T0127614

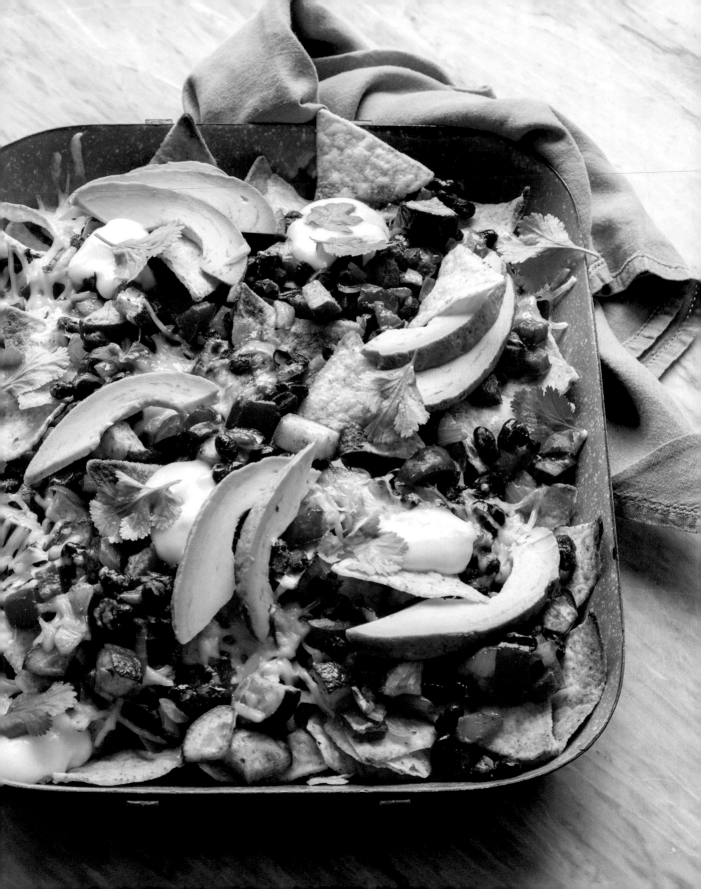

healthy LITTLE TUMMIES

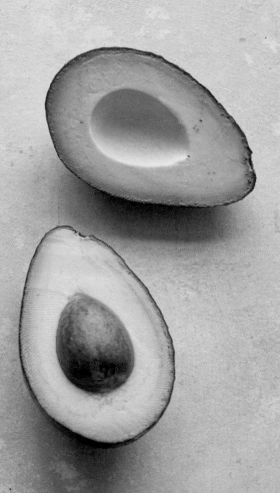

PLANT-BASED
FOOD FOR
THE WHOLE
FAMILY

CLAIRE POWER

WITH PHOTOGRAPHY BY
CLARE WINFIELD

RYLAND PETERS & SMALL
LONDON • NEW YORK

dedication

To my husband and children for always believing in me and supporting me through all my dreams and goals.

Senior editor Miriam Catley
Head of production Patricia Harrington
Art director Leslie Harrington
Editorial director Julia Charles
Publisher Cindy Richards
Indexer Vanessa Bird

Food stylist Maud Eden
Props stylist Olivia Wardle

Published in 2020 by
Ryland Peters & Small
20–21 Jockey's Fields, London
WC1R 4BW and
341 E 116th St, New York
NY 10029

www.rylandpeters.com

10 9 8 7 6 5 4 3 2 1

ISBN: 978-1-78879-234-9

Printed and bound in China

A CIP record for this book is available from the British Library. US Library of Congress CIP data has been applied for.

notes

- Both British (Metric) and Imperial plus US cup measurements are included here for your convenience, however, it is important to work with one set of measurements and not alternate between them within a recipe.
- All spoon measurements are level unless otherwise specified.
- Ovens should be preheated to the specified temperatures. We recommend using an oven thermometer.
- Allergen advice is a guide. Always check food and packaging labels to ensure the food you use is safe for you to consume. If you are following a vegan diet or have an egg allergy you will need to check that the pasta you buy is egg-free, for example.
- Neither the author nor the publisher can be held responsible for any claim arising out of the information in this book. Always consult your health advisor or doctor if you have any concerns about your own or your family's health or nutritional needs.

contents

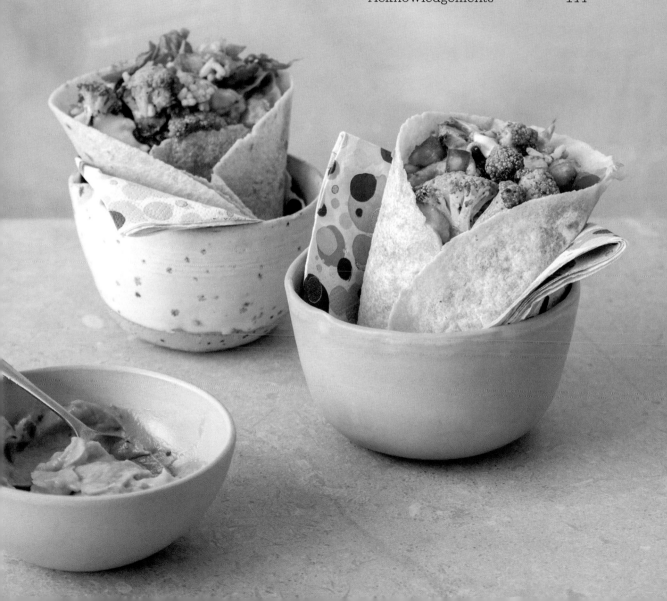

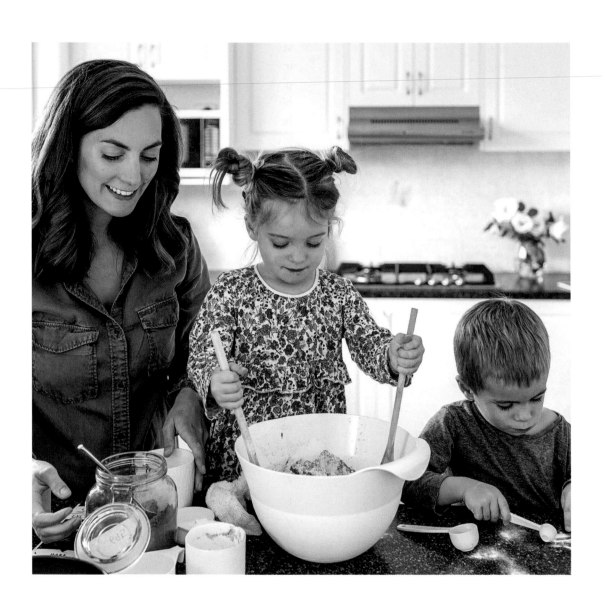

introduction

Hi! I am Claire! I'm a nutritionist and food blogger. Some of you might know me from my recipe blog and website Healthy French Wife where I share healthy plant-based recipes. I'm French/Australian and a mum of three. I have twins called Eloise and James who are 4 years old and Annabelle who is currently 18 months old. All three of them are thriving on a plant-based diet.

A little bit more about myself: I grew up in France and moved to Australia at 18 to study. I fell in love with the country and my now-Australian husband and I stayed in Australia. We lived in Perth for 10 years and moved to Orange, NSW, 2 years ago.

I became vegan after having my twins and the desire to regain my health. I did a 30-day vegan challenge and from then I have stayed vegan for the past 3 years. I loved how eating vegan made me feel, getting more energy, better skin, and better digestion as well as losing a few extra kilos gained during my pregnancy. I have now been vegan for 3 years and I had a successful vegan pregnancy with Annabelle. I am raising predominantly plant-based children and I am very passionate about plant-based nutrition for children and families.

Indeed, I am a qualified nutritionist and I specialize in plant-based nutrition, women's nutrition, pregnancy, and children's nutrition. I became a nutritionist in 2016 after studying Human Nutrition with Deakin University. I also did a health coaching degree shortly after starting my healthy Instagram account in 2013. I found my passion for healthy plant-based food and nutrition through my blog. I love sharing content on social media and helping others live a healthy plant-based lifestyle. I feel very grateful to have been able to turn my passion into my full-time job and now write a healthy, plant-based family cookbook.

Whether you are wanting to increase your intake of plant-based meals or commit to a vegan lifestyle, you will be benefitting the health of your children and yourself by doing so. Through my blog and this cookbook, I hope to help other women and families achieve a more healthy, plant-based lifestyle.

I hope you will find my recipes helpful in sharing plant-based meals as a family, whether your family and children are fully vegan or you are just wanting to eat more plant-based meals and reduce your animal protein consumption. Please remember you don't have to strive for perfection but rather have an overall goal to increase your plant-based meals to improve your health. I hope you will find my recipes delicious and easy to make and they will inspire you to eat more plant-based meals as a family. I encourage you to follow my recipes the first time of making them and make sure to read them fully beforehand, as sometimes they need a little bit of preparation such as soaking nuts ahead of time! Thank you so much for reading my book and happy cooking.

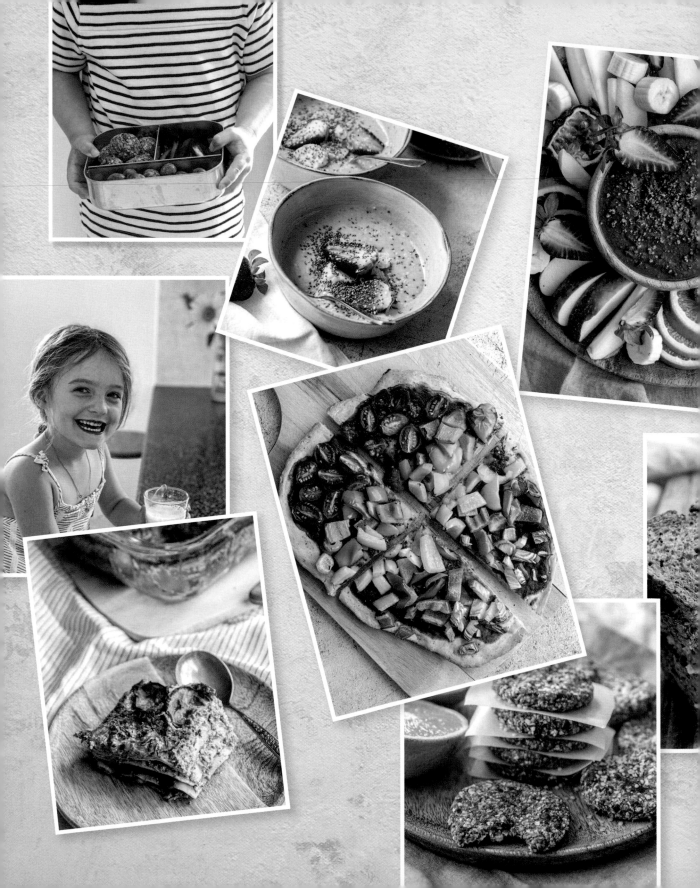

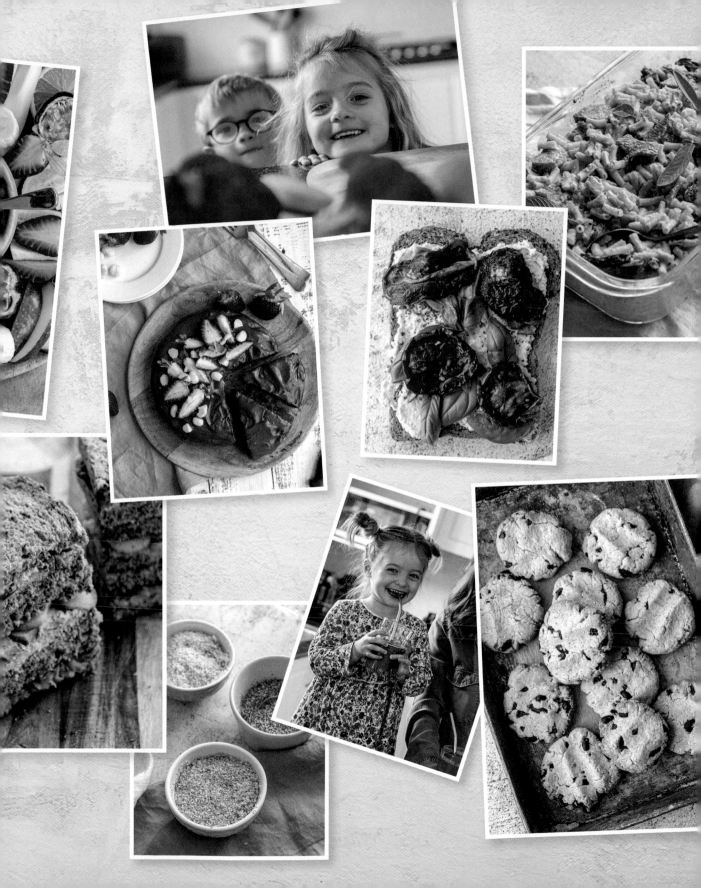

Why choose plant-based?

Following a plant-based diet means eating food that comes from plants and eliminating processed foods as well as animal proteins. It does not always mean being vegan, however, most people eating a plant-based diet choose to be vegan.

Plant-based eating is proven to be the healthiest diet to reduce the risk of common diseases such as cancer, diabetes, obesity and cardiovascular diseases. It is also the most sustainable way to eat for the planet and the environment as well as being kind to animals. Eating a diet rich in plant-foods also helps to improve digestion, skin health and gives you lots of energy.

Choosing to raise children vegan either from birth or making the switch after a few years can benefit their health and reduce their risks of diseases such as diabetes, cardiovascular disease, strokes, obesity and cancer. A vegan or vegetarian diet is recognized as safe and adequate for all ages including toddlers and teenagers by the British Nutrition Foundation, the American Dietary Association and the Dieticians Association of Australia, so long as children eat a well-planned, balanced and varied diet to get all the nutrients they need for proper growth and development.

Nutritional guidelines for children

Based on the British Nutrition Foundation and the Australian Dietary Guidelines, children aged 1–13 are recommended to eat the following every day:

4–5 servings of starchy carbohydrates
1 serving can represent:
• ½–1 slice of bread
• 6 tablespoons breakfast cereal
• 1–3 tablespoons mashed potato
• 2–5 tablespoons cooked pasta/rice

5 servings of fruit and vegetables (at least 4 servings of vegetables and 1–2 servings of fruit)
1 serving can represent:
• ½–1 banana
• 2–3 broccoli florets
• 4–6 carrot sticks
• 1 apple
• 3–10 grapes

3 portions of protein
1 portion can represent:
• 2–4 tablespoons beans, lentils and soya products

2 calcium-rich food servings
1 serving can represent:
• 100 ml/3½ fl. oz./⅓ cup of soya or other fortified plant milks
• 2–4 tablespoons tofu
• 1–2 tablespoons tahini

In addition to these nutritional requirements, I encourage parents to give children healthy fats every day such as ¼–½ avocado, flaxseed meal or flax oil, hemp seeds or hemp oil as well as a range of seeds and nuts.

Every child will have a different appetite, depending on age and food preferences. Appetites can vary from day to day and it's important to offer food from each food group daily and let the child decide how much to eat. Teenagers can be expected to eat 5–7 servings of grains and a higher amount of protein, vegetables and calcium-rich foods than younger children.

Fats, oils and sweet foods should only be used sparingly in a child's diet. Water should be the main drink for your child apart from 1–2 glasses of calcium-fortified plant milks per day in a smoothie or cereals, for example.

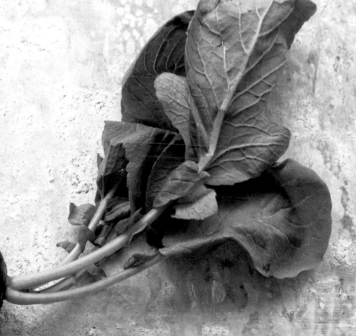

Nutritional tips for eating a healthy plant-based diet

The key to maintaining a healthy plant-based diet in the long-term is to eat a diet of balanced, abundant and diverse plant-based foods. Fill your fridge and plate with whole foods, vegetables, fruits, wholegrains, beans, seeds and nuts. Aiming to reduce processed foods, oils, and refined sugar and refined carbohydrates will help achieve great health for the whole family.

Protein

Eating daily servings of legumes, beans and soya products as well as wholegrains, seeds and nuts, will cover daily protein requirements without the need to supplement with protein powders or animal protein.

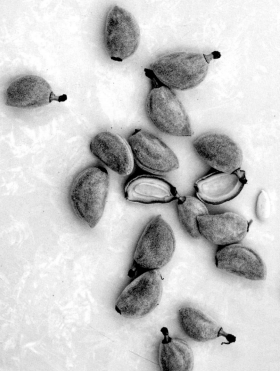

Plant protein sources include:
• Soya (including tofu and tempeh)
• Chickpeas, lentils, beans and peas
• Nuts and nut butters such as cashews, almonds and peanuts
• Chia seeds and hemp seeds
• Sunflower seeds and pumpkin seeds
• Grains such as buckwheat, millet, oats, quinoa and spelt

Carbohydrates

Carbohydrates should represent more than the majority of the macronutrients eaten on a plant-based diet. For a healthy vegan diet, try switching white refined carbohydrates for wholegrains and complex carbohydrates which will not only give you long-lasting energy but also give your body important protein, vitamins and minerals. My favourite carbohydrate sources on a plant-based diet are:
• Brown rice and basmati rice
• Quinoa
• Buckwheat flour and buckwheat pasta
• Wholemeal/whole-wheat pasta
• Starchy vegetables such as sweet potatoes, pumpkin/squash and white potatoes
• Millet
• White pasta and rice (occasionally)

Fats

A healthy plant-based diet should include daily servings of fats especially monounsaturated fat and Omega-6s and Omega-3s. I recommend focusing on wholefood fat sources such as seeds, avocado and nuts and reducing processed foods and oils to achieve this.

Oils are caloric-dense and nutrient-poor as well as being highly processed and often too high in omega-6s, the cause of inflammation in the body, and saturated fats (especially coconut oil) which raise cholesterol and is the cause of cardiovascular disease. I recommend using vegetable oils and coconut oil sparingly or not at all. Extra virgin olive oil, avocado oil and flaxseed oil are healthier oils to consume cold. Olive oil and organic cold-pressed canola/rapeseed oil are best to use when cooking, or try cooking oil-free by sautéing vegetables in water.

Tahini, avocado, hemp seeds and Brazil nuts should be eaten regularly especially for children on a plant-based diet.

Omega-3s

Omega-3s, or Alpha Linoleic Acid (ALA), are essential fatty acids that our body requires for a healthy immune system as well as optimal eye and brain function. The body can transform ALA into eicosapentaenoic acid (EPA) and docosahexaenoic acid (DHA).

Eating enough Omega-3s can require a little bit more planning on a vegan diet, but Omega-3 daily requirements can be achieved by consuming flaxseed meal or ground linseed, chia seeds, hemp seeds and walnuts and,

if required, through an algae supplement for children not eating enough of the other sources of Omega-3s.

Getting the right balance of Omega-3s and Omega-6s is also really important. Eating too many Omega-6s such as sunflower oil, seeds and vegetable oils can reduce your body's ability to convert ALA into EPA and DHA. Eating a well-planned wholefood plant-based diet can help achieve the desirable Omega-3 to Omega-6 ratio of about one to four.

I use a lot of flaxseed meal and hemp seeds in my recipes and these are two essential ingredients that I use daily for my family and myself. I love the nutty taste of both flaxseed meal and hemp seeds and they add a healthy dose of Omega-3s, protein and fibre into our diet. Flaxseed meal is also great for baking to act as an egg replacement. I recommend storing your flaxseed meal and hemp seeds in the fridge to avoid them going rancid.

Calcium

Calcium is needed for strong bones and teeth. Children need a lot of calcium for healthy bone development. Young children require 700mg of calcium daily and older children 1000mg. Teenagers require 1300mg daily. Calcium found in plant-based foods is well absorbed, but to reach requirements it is recommended to eat calcium-rich foods such as tofu, soya milk, tahini, leafy greens (kale/collard greens, bok choy/pak choi), broccoli, almonds and almond butter, calcium-fortified orange juice and calcium-fortified plant milks. Did you know calcium-fortified plant milks contain as much calcium as cow's milk?

Iron

Iron is used by our bodies to transport oxygen to our muscles and organs and is important for keeping us energized and our moods stable. Iron needs are a lot higher for women generally: women aged 19–50 (14.8mg), menstruating girls (18mg) and pregnant women (27mg). Children need between 8–11mg per day depending on their age. Children should eat a variety of foods that contain iron every day. Infants should be introduced to iron-rich foods as soon as they start on solid foods at around six months of age such as iron-fortified rice cereals. If children do not meet their iron requirements they may develop iron-deficiency anaemia.

Daily iron requirements are easily attainable when eating an abundant and balanced plant-based diet that contains many sources of non-haem iron. Foods that contain non-haem iron include:
• Wholegrain bread and cereals
• Iron-fortified breakfast cereals
• Legumes including baked beans, dried peas, beans, lentils
• Green leafy vegetables
• Dried fruit
• Peanut butter

Iron absorption is increased 2–3-fold when eating a meal containing iron-rich foods along with vitamin-C rich fruits or vegetables such as (bell) peppers/capsicums, broccoli, kiwi fruits or citrus fruits. Avoiding caffeine in the form of coffee and tea around mealtimes also helps with improving your body's ability to absorb iron. I recommend getting iron levels checked by a blood test and see your doctor if you are showing signs of deficiency or if you are worried that your child might be deficient.

Vitamin B12

Vitamin B12 is very important for red blood cell formation, brain and nervous system function and DNA replication. Deficiencies in vitamin B12 can be dangerous and lead to tiredness and illness.

Vitamin B12 is created by bacteria found in the soil and sadly, due to over-farming and over-washing vegetables, vitamin 12 is not available in plant-based foods. Even livestock have to be supplemented with vitamin B12.

Vegan sources of vitamin B12 include foods that are fortified with vitamin B12, some soya milks, nutritional yeast (more on nutritional yeast, below) and some vegetarian meat such as soya-based burgers and sausages.

I recommending supplementing with a quality vitamin B12 supplement if you aren't consuming many food sources. You can find vitamin B12 in sprays to use with children. It's a good idea to get your levels checked by your GP once a year.

A note on fortified nutritional yeast: I use these yellow flakes in a lot of my savoury recipes. They are a must to make cheesy-like sauces and creams in vegan dishes. I even sprinkle some on my salads and to top pasta dishes. Nutritional yeast is also very good for you. It contains vitamin B12, fibre, protein, B vitamins and minerals. You can find it in most supermarkets or in health food shops.

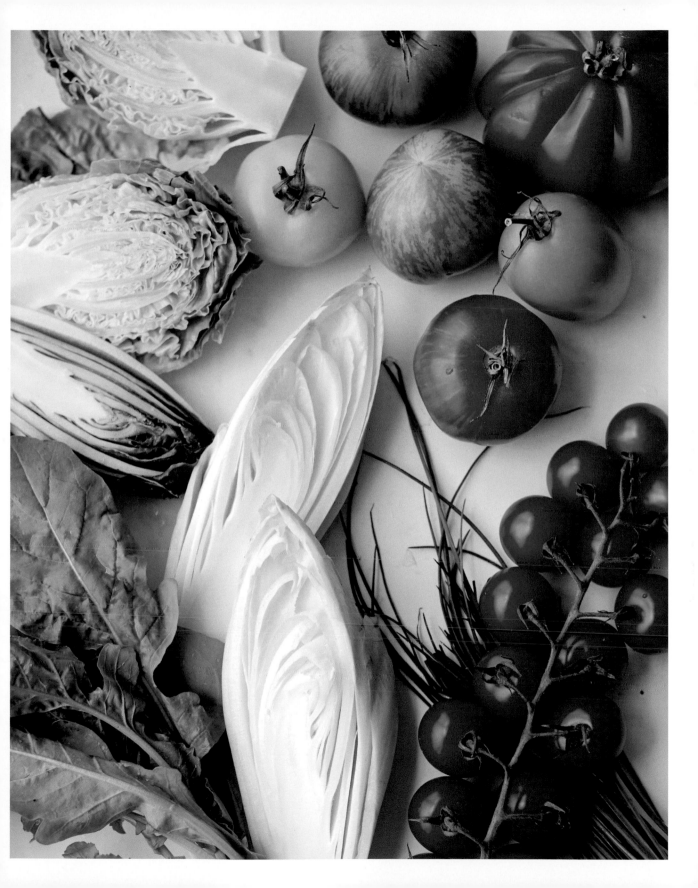

Getting started

Transitioning to a plant-based diet can seem daunting and difficult with children, but it is very achievable and without noticing you have probably fed them a lot of vegan meals in the past. A lot of children's favourite foods are already vegan such as fruit and chips. Here are some tips to get started:

Start with one plant-based meal a day

Some people decide to go vegan completely overnight, others prefer to ease into it. Swapping one meal per day to plant-based is a great way to transition. Breakfast, for example, is easy to transition by switching dairy for plant-based milks, making smoothies, granolas, avocado toasts or one of the breakfast recipes in this cookbook.

Get your family involved

Children love to get involved with cooking, planning meals and shopping for food. It can help them embrace this new lifestyle. Why not pick a few recipes together in this cookbook that you would like to make, then shop and cook the meals together?

Fill your fridge and pantry

Plant-based eating does not mean eating weird and wonderful ingredients. I aim to only use familiar ingredients in my recipes. I do my shopping at the main supermarkets and local market or grocer. I sometimes buy a few ingredients from a health food shop, too. I find since being vegan our food budget is half of what it used to be!

Vegetables

Vegetables should be the bulk of your food shopping. Aim to buy seasonal vegetables, where possible. My go-to vegetables to buy every week include:
- Broccoli, cauliflower, spinach, red cabbage
- Courgettes/zucchinis, (bell) peppers/capsicums
- Carrots, onions, garlic, spring onions/scallions
- Cos lettuce, avocados, cucumber, tomatoes
- Pumpkin/squash, sweet potatoes, potatoes

Fruits

I recommend stocking up on a wide range of in-season fruits every week. Bananas, oranges, berries and apples are staples in our home. We always have a very large fruit basket on the kitchen counter and when my kids are hungry they can grab a piece of fruit. I also like cutting some fruit and serving it as a fruit platter for an afternoon snack.

Pantry

My storecupboard essentials include:
- Canned beans, lentils and chickpeas
- Chickpea/gram flour
- Wholemeal/whole-wheat flour
- Pasta (wholemeal/whole-wheat or buckwheat)
- Rice (basmati or brown rice)
- Quinoa
- Canned tomatoes
- Nutritional yeast
- Oats
- Maple syrup/coconut sugar
- Canned coconut milk and coconut cream
- Seeds and nuts including hemp seeds, chia seeds, flaxseeds, almonds, cashews, walnuts, Brazil nuts and peanuts
- Olive oil and coconut oil

Spices and herbs

Good-quality spices and herbs are very important to cook delicious vegan meals. I always have the following on my shelves:

• Garlic, onion and curry powder
• Ground cumin, cinnamon, paprika, turmeric
• Garam masala
• Dried Italian herbs
• Salt and freshly ground black pepper

Equipment

I don't have much fancy kitchen equipment, but I do recommend a good-quality, high-speed food processor/blender.

A note on food allergies

My little girl Annabelle had some infant food allergies. For the first 12 months of her life she was allergic to soya and wheat so I understand how difficult dealing with food allergies or having a child with food allergies can be. All my recipes are egg-free **EF** and dairy-free **DF** and some are also soya-free **SYF**, nut-free **NF** and gluten-free **GF**.

Each recipe will have allergy labels. However, always check the ingredients list when using store-bought products such as sauces, pastas and chocolate.

OF Oil-free:
I have also included the label oil-free as I like to keep our family's oil-consumption low, and as such, I have created some oil-free recipes. My tip for cooking oil-free is to use a little bit of water instead of oil when cooking in a pan and adding flavour using spices and herbs.

SYF Soya-free:
Most of my recipes are soya-free. My little girl had an infant allergy to soya so I know first-hand how hard it is to be vegan and soya-free. I have used tofu and tamari in some recipes, both of which contain soya. You can substitute the tofu for beans and the tamari with coconut aminos to make those recipes soya-free.

NF Nut-free:
I have created a lot of nut-free recipes, but you can also make most recipes nut-free by substituting cashew cheese sauce for store-bought vegan cheese and using seeds instead of nuts in other recipes. Sunflower seeds and sunflower butter are a great substitute for peanuts and peanut butter.

GF Gluten-free:
If the recipe is not already gluten-free you can easily make it so by substituting gluten-free oats or quinoa flakes and using gluten-free flours and pasta. When baking gluten-free, I recommend using a quality one-to-one gluten-free flour blend.

WF Wheat-free:
Some of my recipes might include sources of gluten but no wheat. My go-to wheat-free grains are oats, barley and rye, as well as those that are also gluten-free, such as quinoa, amaranth, teff and buckwheat.

SF Sugar-free:
All my recipes are refined-sugar-free but I use maple syrup and coconut sugar in sweet recipes.

I hope this cookbook can help you in your journey towards a healthy plant-based lifestyle. Feel free to tag me @healthyfrenchwife on Instagram or use #healthylittletummies so I can see your posts and stories.

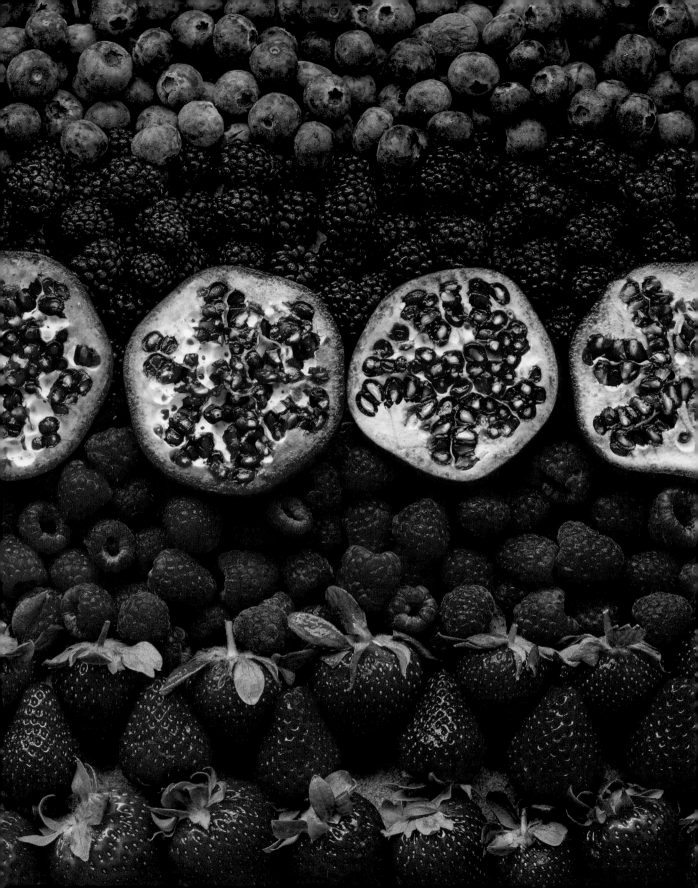

BREAKFAST

berry hemp smoothie

chocolate granola

breakfast strawberry yogurt bowl

raw buckwheat porridge

blueberry muffins

apple coconut bircher

homemade date & hemp seed muesli

vegan buckwheat coconut pancakes

abc nut butter

chocolate hazelnut spread

berry hemp smoothie

Drinking this smoothie is a very nutritious way to start the day. Feel free to use strawberries or blueberries or frozen berries, too. Hemp seeds are my favourite seeds as they are such a nutritious seed – high in protein, iron and omega-3 and perfect for kids on a plant-based diet. I also like adding one vegetable to our smoothies, such as baby spinach, raw cauliflower or courgette/zucchini, as well as 1 tablespoon of nut butter or tahini and seeds for protein and good fats, to make our smoothies filling enough and to give us energy to last all morning.

1 banana
350 g/12 oz. fresh or frozen
  berries of choice
375 ml/1½ cups oat milk
20 g/½ cup baby spinach or raw
  courgette/zucchini
2 tablespoons hemp seeds
1 tablespoon tahini
½ teaspoon ground cinnamon
1–2 pitted medjool dates for
  sweetness (optional)

SERVES 2–3

PREP TIME: 5 MINUTES

In a blender, combine all the ingredients and blend on high until smooth.

Add the dates, if desired, blend and serve.

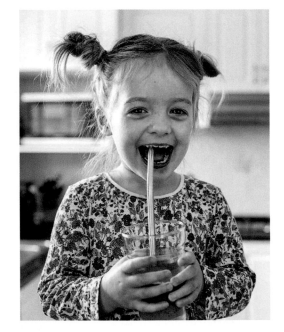

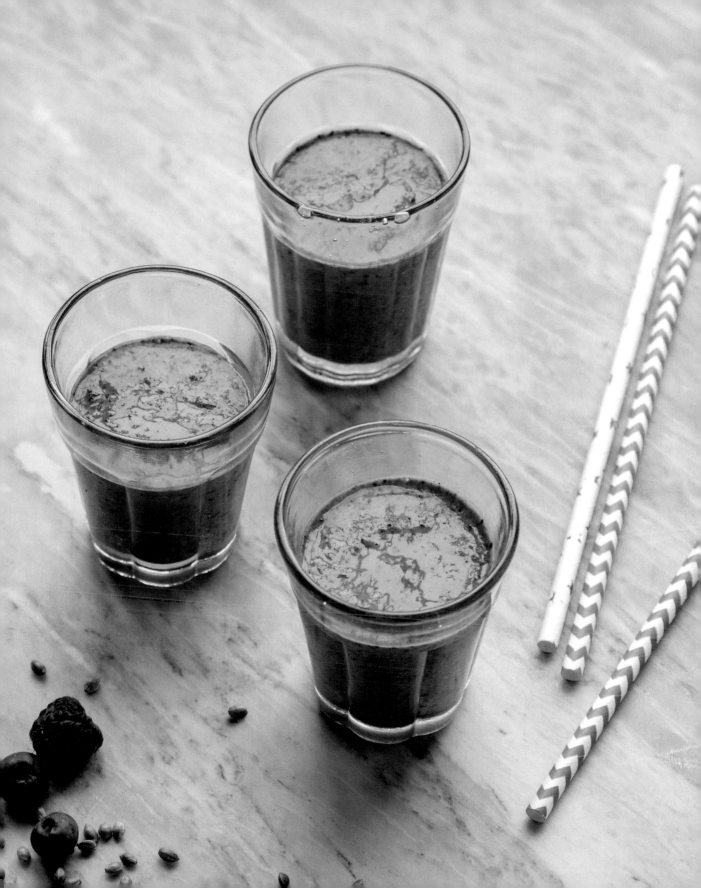

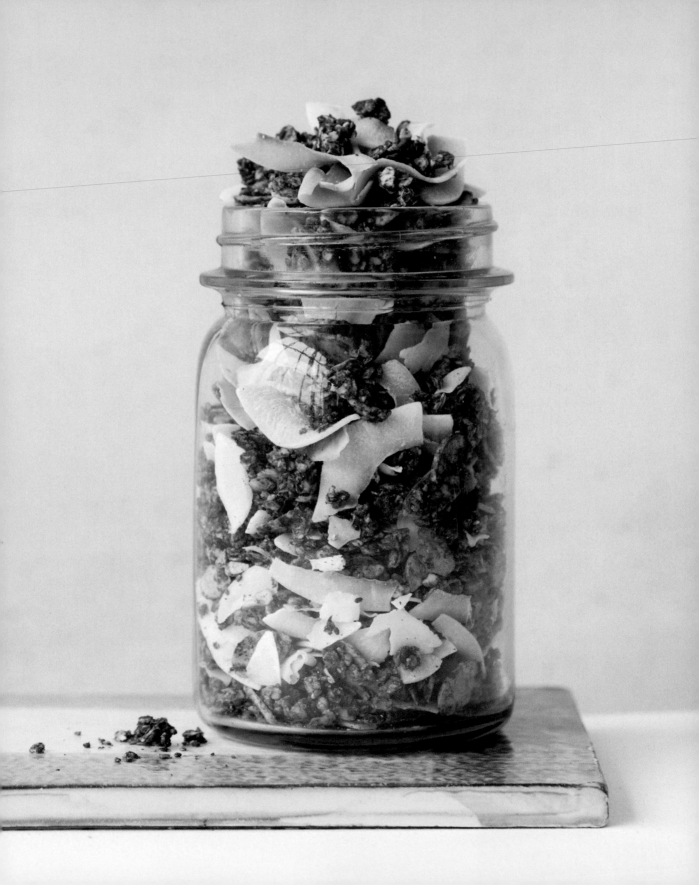

chocolate granola

This chocolate granola makes us excited to wake up and have breakfast! It is absolutely delicious served with cold plant milk, to snack on or with a bowl of coconut yogurt and berries. It is also a lot healthier than store-bought granolas and very easy to make. The only issue is that it disappears too quickly when I make it!

200 g/2 cups rolled/old-fashioned oats
100 g/1 cup desiccated/dried shredded coconut or dried coconut flakes
60 g/⅓ cup chia seeds
30 g/⅓ cup raw cacao powder
125 ml/½ cup melted coconut oil
2 tablespoons maple syrup
flaked/slivered almonds (optional)

baking sheet lined with parchment paper

SERVES 6–8

PREP TIME: 5 MINUTES
COOKING TIME: 20–25 MINUTES

Preheat the oven to 180°C (350°F) Gas 4.

In a mixing bowl, mix all of the ingredients together and stir with a spoon until well combined.

Spread out the granola evenly on the prepared baking sheet and bake it in the preheated oven for 20–25 minutes.

Leave to cool on the baking sheet before breaking into granola clusters.

Variations: Add nuts, seeds, grated orange zest, dried fruits.

breakfast strawberry yogurt bowl

This simple breakfast option is packed with protein and calcium and can be made the night before. I often struggle finding good dairy-free vegan yogurts that are natural and not full of sugar or weird ingredients, which is why I made this so-called 'yogurt' using silken tofu by blending it with strawberries. You can enjoy it with granola, fruit, seeds or on its own. I have tried it with mango in summer and it is amazing.

300 g/10½ oz. silken tofu
125 g/1¼ cups fresh strawberries
2 tablespoons maple syrup
1 teaspoon vanilla extract

SERVES 2–3

PREP TIME: 5 MINUTES

In a blender, combine the ingredients together and blend until smooth. Serve in two or three bowls and top with fruit, seeds, nuts and/or granola.

Store in an airtight container in the fridge for up to 3 days.

Variations: You can substitute the strawberries for blueberries, raspberries, mango, peaches or passion fruit. Top with granola or fruit, add chia seeds, hemp seeds or nuts.

DF EF GF WF
NF OF

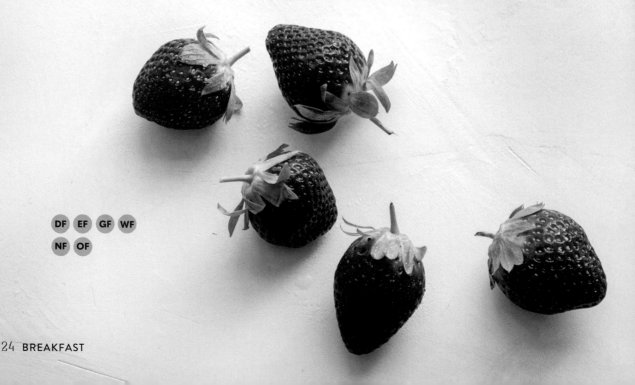

raw buckwheat porridge

We have oatmeal porridge most days for breakfast, especially in winter, so it is nice to make a different porridge. If you have never tried buckwheat it is one of my favourite gluten-free seeds. I love using the flour in baking and the buckwheat groats make for a nutritious breakfast. This recipe takes a little bit more work as you have to soak the groats overnight, but it can be made quite quickly in the morning. You can play around by using different plant milks, nut butter, berries or raw cacao powder.

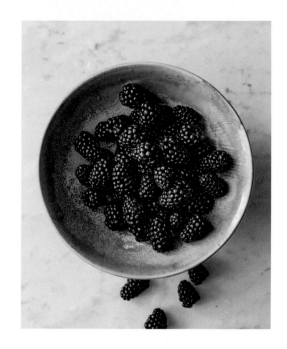

400 g/2 cups buckwheat groats
250 ml/1 cup plant milk of choice
60 ml/¼ cup maple syrup
2 tablespoons flaxseed meal
1 teaspoon ground cinnamon
1 teaspoon vanilla essence
150–300 g/1–2 cups frozen
    or fresh berries

SERVES 4–6

**PREP TIME: 2–3 HOURS
(INCLUDING SOAKING TIME)**

Soak the buckwheat groats in water for 2–3 hours or overnight, then drain and rinse very well.

Add the buckwheat groats to a blender or food processor along with the remaining ingredients including the berries and blend to combine. Don't over-process it – aim to keep a bit of texture.

Divide the porridge between bowls and serve. Store leftovers in the fridge for up to 2–3 days in an airtight container.

blueberry muffins

My son James loves blueberries and baked goods so I like making these muffins for him to have as a treat sometimes. I use coconut sugar which gives them a darker colour. You could swap the blueberries for any other berries (fresh or frozen) and you could top them with chocolate chips, chopped nuts and/or seeds. If you wanted to make them gluten-free I would recommend swapping the self-raising/rising wholemeal/whole-wheat flour with the equivalent in buckwheat flour and adding 2 teaspoons of baking powder, or using a self-raising/rising gluten-free flour baking blend.

300 g/2 cups self-raising/rising
   wholemeal/whole-wheat flour
½ teaspoon ground cinnamon
120 g/¾ cup coconut sugar
250 ml/1 cup plant milk of choice
125 ml/½ cup melted coconut oil
   or olive oil
120 g/1 cup frozen blueberries
1 tablespoon flaxseed meal
blueberries and mixed seeds
   (optional)

12-hole muffin pan lined with
   muffin cases

MAKES 12 MUFFINS

PREP TIME: 5 MINUTES
COOKING TIME: 25 MINUTES

Preheat the oven to 180°C (350°F) Gas 4.

In a mixing bowl, combine the flour, cinnamon and coconut sugar. Add in the plant milk and stir to combine with a spoon. Pour the melted coconut or olive oil into the bowl and combine further with a spoon. Add the frozen berries and fold gently into the dough with a spatula. Do not over stir.

Spoon the batter into the muffin cases filling each about halfway to the top, and top with additional blueberries and/or mixed seeds, if using.

Put the muffins into the preheated oven and bake for 25 minutes until lightly golden. Remove from the oven and transfer to a wire rack to cool.

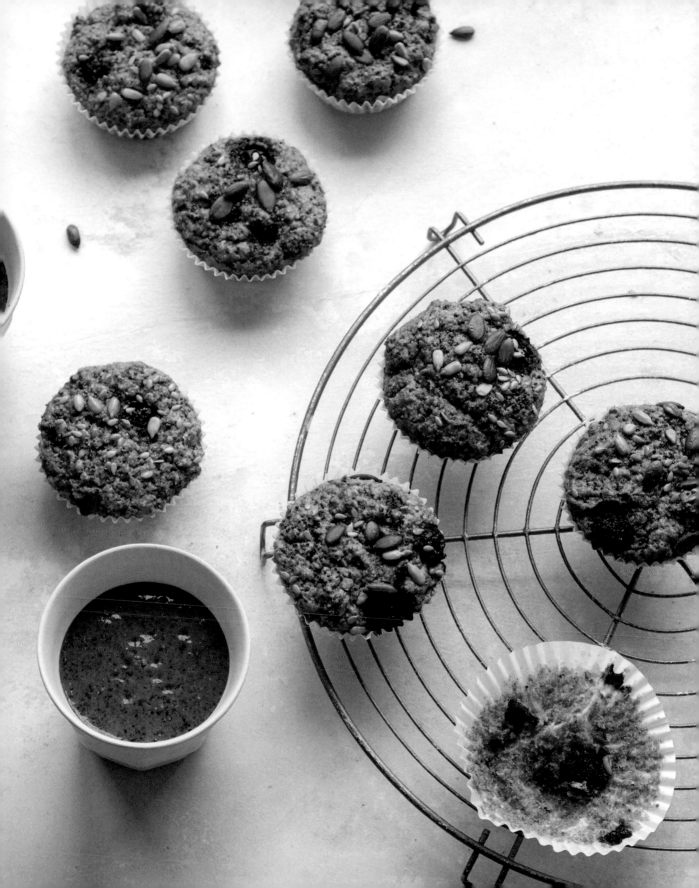

apple coconut bircher

My kids and I are big fans of bircher muesli for breakfast. I love it even more as a busy mum of three as it can be made the night before. I like this apple and coconut combination, but we sometimes swap the grated apples for frozen raspberries, diced mango or peaches in summer.

2 medium apples, cored
  and grated
200 g/2 cups gluten-free rolled/
  old-fashioned oats
625 ml/2½ cups coconut milk,
  plus extra to serve
30 g/½ cup desiccated coconut
2 tablespoons chia seeds
1 teaspoon ground cinnamon
coconut yogurt, to serve (optional)

SERVES 4–6

**PREP TIME: 10 MINUTES
AND OVERNIGHT SOAKING TIME**

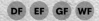

In a mixing bowl, combine all the ingredients together and place in the fridge to soak overnight.

Serve with a splash of coconut milk or coconut yogurt, if desired.

Variations: Use frozen berries, coconut yogurt, peaches, mangoes, almond milk, maple syrup, sliced bananas, nuts, and/or seeds.

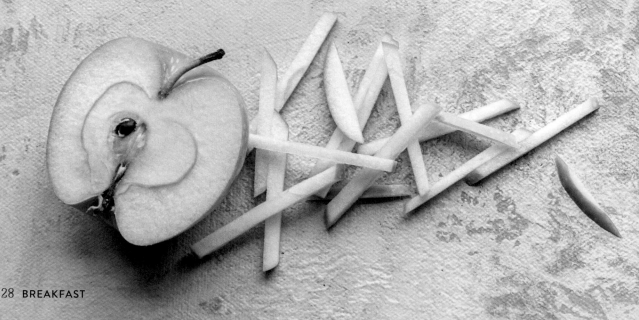

homemade date & hemp seed muesli

Making your own muesli is a great way to avoid store-bought cereals packed with sugar, preservatives, vegetable oils and other weird ingredients. I love using this muesli with cold plant milk or warm oat milk for a warm porridge in winter. If you do not have hemp seeds, you can swap them for sunflower or pumpkin seeds or crushed nuts. The dates make this sweet enough to have on its own.

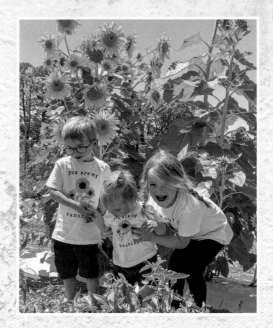

70 g/½ cup pitted dates
100 g/1 cup desiccated/dried
  shredded coconut
200 g/2 cups gluten-free rolled/
  old-fashioned oats
65 g/½ cup hemp seeds
½ teaspoon ground cinnamon

SERVES 4

PREP TIME: 5 MINUTES

In a food processor combine all the ingredients together and pulse a few times until the oats and dates are chopped into smaller pieces. Do not over-process, keep it chunky.

Serve with hot or cold plant milk and your favourite fruit.

DF EF GF WF
NF OF SF SYF

vegan buckwheat coconut pancakes

I love starting our Sundays with a batch of these fluffy wholegrain vegan pancakes. They often make an appearance on special mornings such as birthdays and Mother's Day breakfast. We love topping them with sliced banana, blueberries and maple syrup or coconut yogurt.

150 g/1 cup buckwheat flour
1 teaspoon baking powder
1 teaspoon vanilla essence
375 ml/1½ cups coconut milk
olive oil or coconut oil spray,
    for cooking
fruit and maple syrup or vegan
    caramel sauce, to top

MAKES 10 SMALL PANCAKES

PREP TIME: 5–10 MINUTES
COOKING TIME: 10–15 MINUTES

In a mixing bowl, combine the buckwheat flour, baking powder and vanilla essence.

Add the coconut milk and whisk to combine, taking care to remove any lumps.

Heat a frying pan/skillet over a medium heat, spray the pan with olive oil or coconut oil spray, and pour 60 ml/ ¼ cup of the pancake batter into the hot pan. Leave to cook for a few minutes or until bubbles have formed on the surface then flip and cook the other side for around 1–2 minutes.

Remove to a plate and keep warm. Repeat with the remaining batter and serve the pancakes with the topping of your choice.

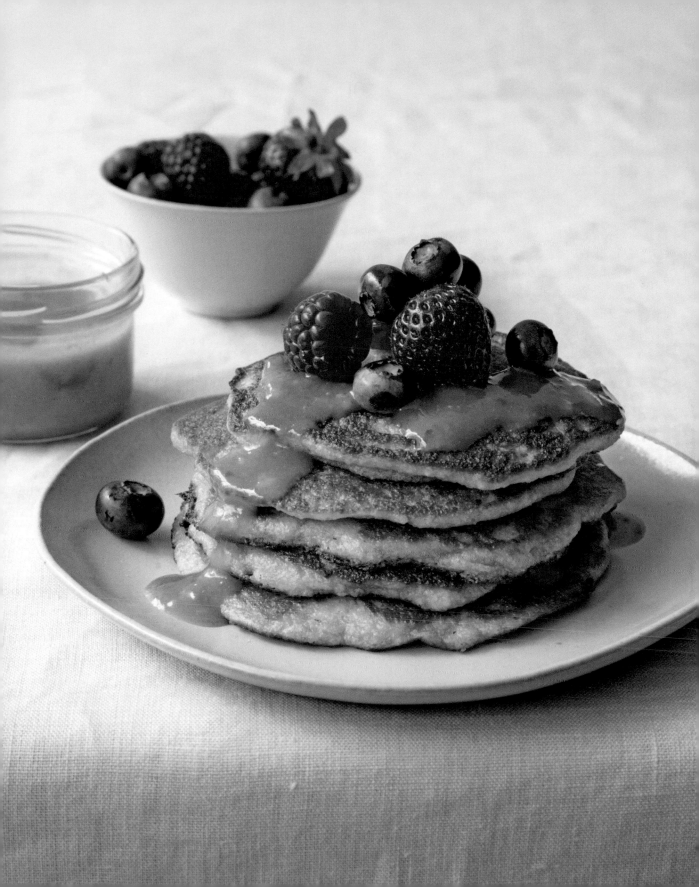

I grew up on the popular non-vegan chocolate spread and am glad my children do not have to miss out with this super delicious and healthy chocolate hazelnut spread. ABC nut butter is made with almonds, Brazil nuts and cashew nuts. You can change up the quantities based on what you have in your pantry. Great to spread on wholemeal toast, served with fruit to dip or simply by the spoon!

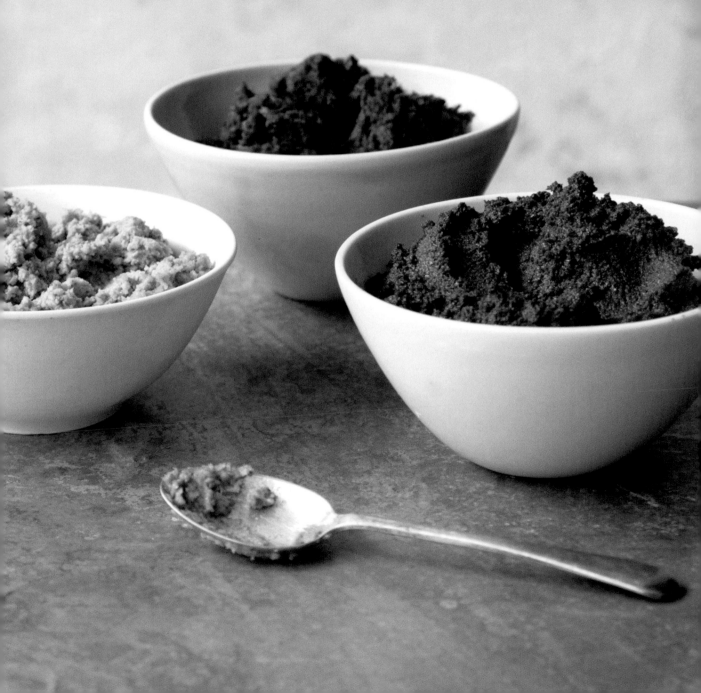

chocolate hazelnut spread

150 g/1 cup raw hazelnuts
60 ml/¼ cup maple syrup
3 tablespoons raw cacao powder
1 teaspoon vanilla essence

baking sheet, lined with parchment paper

MAKES 1 JAR OF AROUND 200 G/2 CUPS

PREP TIME: 15 MINUTES
COOK TIME: 10 MINUTES

Preheat the oven to 180°C (350°F) Gas 4.

Put the hazelnuts with their skins onto the prepared baking sheet and roast in the preheated oven for 10 minutes.

Leave the hazelnuts to cool before removing the skins using your hands or rubbing them with a paper towel.

Put the roasted hazelnuts, maple syrup, raw cacao powder, vanilla and 2 tablespoons water in a high-speed blender or food processor and blend for a few minutes or until smooth and creamy.

Put in a sealed jar and enjoy. Store in the fridge for up to 2 weeks.

Variation: Swap hazelnuts for almonds or peanuts for a different nut spread.

abc nut butter

160 g/1 cup raw almonds
70 g/½ cup raw Brazil nuts
70 g/½ cup raw cashews

MAKES ABOUT 250 G/2 CUPS OF NUT BUTTER

PREP TIME: 5 MINUTES

In a high-speed blender or food processor, blend all the nuts together for a few minutes until smooth and creamy. Scrape the side of the blender if needed. It might take a few minutes if your blender is not that powerful.

Store the nut butter in a sealed jar in the fridge for up to 2 weeks.

Variations: Add cinnamon, sea salt, maple syrup or raw cacao powder after blending.

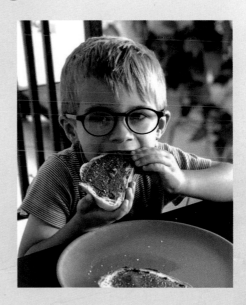

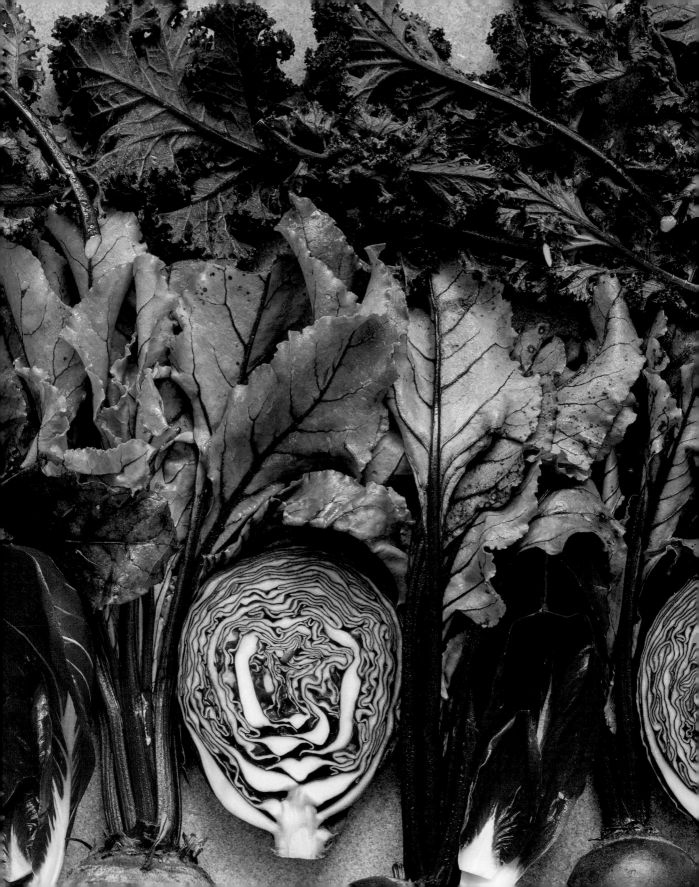

LUNCH

lentil bites

lentil & pumpkin sausage rolls

sweet potato bites

chickpea nuggets

hummus sandwiches 3 ways

pitta sandwiches

chickpea 'omelettes'

spinach & cashew 'ricotta' sausage rolls

pesto wholemeal scrolls

cauliflower burritos

courgette chia meatless balls

lentil bites

These lentil bites are very easy to make and use ingredients that you probably have in your pantry. They are perfect for topping pasta, crumbled in wraps or in salad bowls and lunchboxes.

1 x 420-g/15-oz. can lentils,
   drained and rinsed
60 g/½ cup gluten-free oats
   or quinoa flakes
1 tablespoon tomato purée/paste
1 tablespoon flaxseed meal
1 teaspoon dried Italian herbs

baking sheet lined with parchment
   paper

MAKES 14

PREP TIME: 5 MINUTES
COOKING TIME: 20–25 MINUTES

Preheat the oven to 180°C (350°F) Gas 4.

In a blender or food processor, combine the lentils, oats, tomato purée/paste, flaxseed meal and dried Italian herbs and pulse a few times until it becomes sticky but remains a little chunky.

Roll the mixture into 14 even-sized balls and place them on the prepared baking sheet.

Bake in the preheated oven for 20–25 minutes.

Eat warm or cold, with pasta, crumbled in a sandwich or as a snack for dipping.

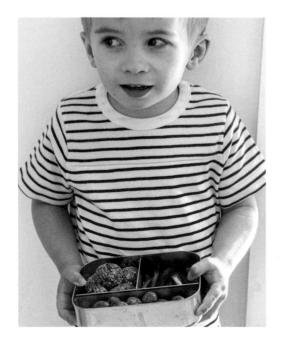

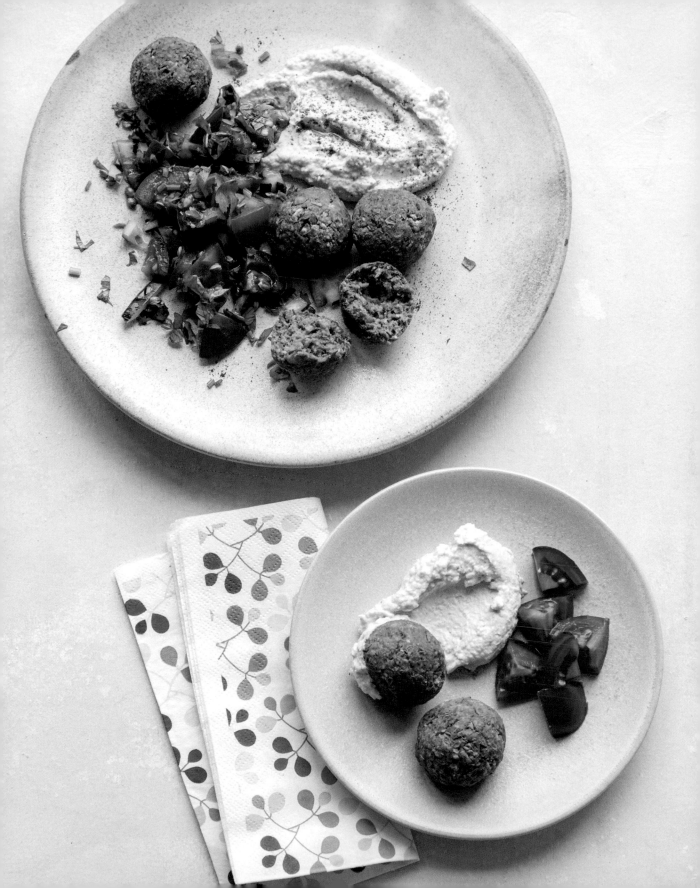

lentil & pumpkin 'sausage' rolls

These healthy vegan 'sausage' rolls will make a great share plate, lunch or light dinner. I often double the quantity as we love them so much! Packed with plant protein, fibre and delicious pumpkin they are really the healthiest 'sausage' rolls. My tip is to make them the day you have leftover roasted pumpkin, prep the pumpkin ahead of time or use canned mashed pumpkin if available where you live. You could add curry powder, kale, spinach or vegan cheese, too. You can use gluten-free pastry sheets to make them gluten-free.

DF EF
NF OF SF

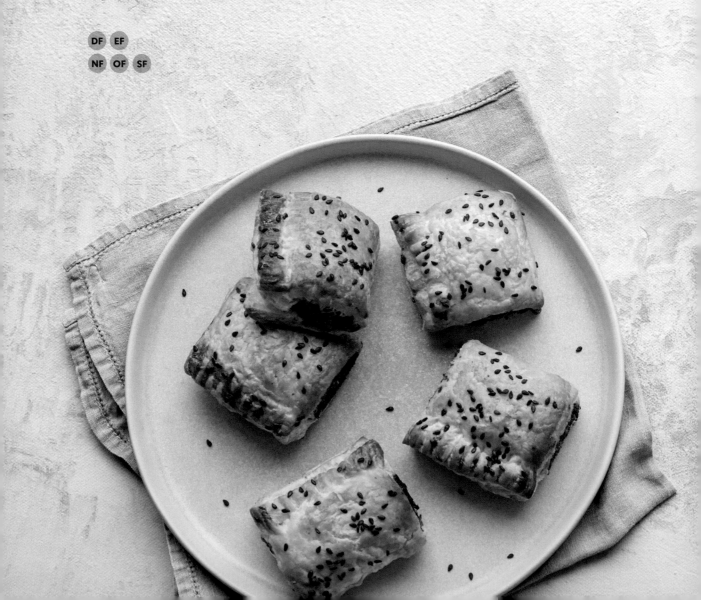

¼ Kent or kabocha pumpkin,
  peeled and deseeded or
  280 g/1 cup mashed pumpkin
2 sheets frozen vegan puff pastry
1 x 420-g/15-oz. can lentils,
  drained and rinsed
60 g/½ cup quick-cook oats
3 tablespoons flaxseed meal
2 tablespoons tomato purée/paste
1 teaspoon sea salt
1 teaspoon onion powder
1 teaspoon ground cumin
1 tablespoon soya milk
1 tablespoon black sesame seeds

*baking sheet lined with parchment
  paper*

MAKES 12

**PREP TIME: 10 MINUTES
COOKING TIME: 20–25 MINUTES
PLUS 39 MINUTES IF USING RAW
PUMPKIN**

Preheat the oven to 200°C (400°F) Gas 6.

If using raw pumpkin, slice the pumpkin and place on the prepared baking sheet. Bake in the preheated oven for 30 minutes.

Defrost the frozen puff pastry sheets.

When the pumpkin is baked, remove from the oven. Mash the pumpkin with a fork in a small bowl.

Combine the mashed pumpkin in a large bowl with the lentils. Add the oats, flaxseed meal, tomato purée/paste, salt and spices and combine well.

Once the pastry sheets are fully defrosted, layer half of the pumpkin mixture onto each pastry sheet to form a sausage-shaped log in the middle.

Gently roll up the 'sausage' rolls tightly enclosing the filling. Brush some soya milk on top, then slice into 3–4-cm/1¼–1½-inch wide sausage rolls.

Place them onto the cleaned, re-lined baking sheet, spaced apart. Sprinkle the sesame seeds on top and bake in the preheated oven for 20–25 minutes until lightly golden.

Serve hot or warm with tomato sauce.

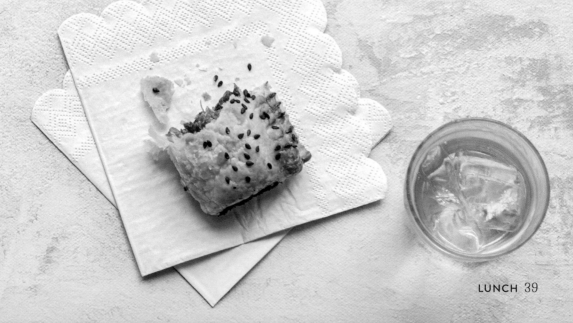

sweet potato bites

When my youngest daughter was a toddler her favourite food was sweet potato bites from a packet. They were pretty expensive and not the healthiest so I decided to make my own version. These would be great for young children learning to eat on their own or even school-aged children to pack in lunch boxes or older children and adults to snack on. I have also made them for picnics and road trips as they are the perfect finger food. If you do not have hemp seeds you can use almond meal instead.

2 medium-sized sweet potatoes
   (about 580 g/20 oz.)
120 g/1 cup oat flour
3 tablespoons hemp seeds
2 tablespoons oat milk
1 tablespoon nutritional yeast
1 teaspoon baking powder
1 teaspoon garlic powder
1 teaspoon ground cumin
½ teaspoon dried Italian herbs
salt and pepper

*baking sheet lined with parchment
   paper*

MAKES 15

PREP TIME: 40 MINUTES
COOKING TIME: 20 MINUTES

Preheat the oven to 180°C (350°F) Gas 4.

Peel and dice the sweet potatoes, place on the lined baking sheet and bake in the preheated oven for 30–40 minutes.

In a blender, combine the diced, baked sweet potato and all the remaining ingredients until completely smooth.

Wet your hands with water and roll the mixture into a long sausage shape, then cut into 2.5-cm/1-inch chunks. Transfer to the clean, re-lined baking sheet and bake in the preheated oven for 15 minutes. Remove from the oven and allow to cool before serving.

Variations: Use buckwheat flour instead of oat flour, curry powder instead of cumin, or add some chopped kale or spinach.

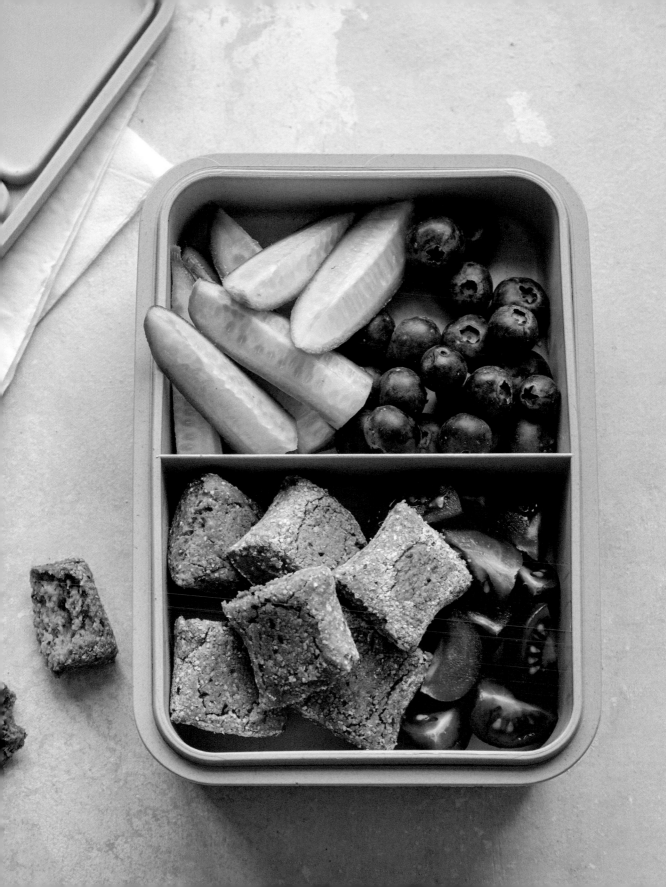

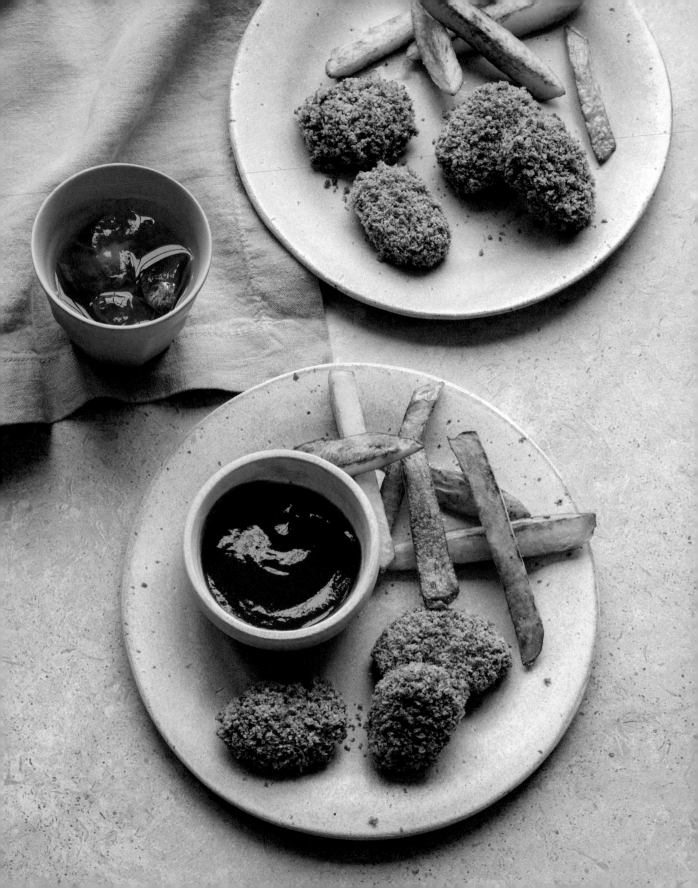

chickpea nuggets

Well before I became vegan, I stopped eating chicken nuggets and I never had the desire to turn to faux-meat vegan nuggets, but when I heard of chickpea nuggets, I knew it was something that I wanted to try to make for my kids. Made with wholesome natural ingredients, it is a fun recipe to share with kids. To make them gluten-free, use gluten-free oats and make the crumbs using quinoa flakes or gluten free breadcrumbs. Store them in an airtight container and reheat in the oven or sandwich presser.

1 x 420-g/15-oz. can chickpeas, drained and rinsed
40 g/⅓ cup rolled/old-fashioned oats
2 tablespoons flax seeds
1–2 tablespoons oat milk
1 teaspoon onion powder
½ teaspoon garlic powder
½ teaspoon dried Italian herbs
pinch of salt and pepper

CRUMBS
60 g/½ cup wholemeal/whole-wheat breadcrumbs
125 ml/½ cup oat milk

baking sheet lined with parchment paper

MAKES 15

PREP TIME: 5 MINUTES
COOKING TIME: 10–15 MINUTES

Preheat the oven to 190°C (375°F) Gas 5.

Put the chickpeas into a food processor or high-speed blender. Add the oats, flax seeds, oat milk, onion and garlic powder, dried herbs and salt and pepper and pulse to blend until well combined and the chickpeas are finely chopped. Do not overblend.

For the outer crumbs, put the breadcrumbs or quinoa flakes and oat milk into two separate small bowls. Shape the chickpea dough into 15 even-size nuggets. Dip each nugget, one at a time, into the milk, then into the breadcrumbs, coating both sides and then put each one onto the prepared baking sheet.

Bake in the preheated oven for 10–15 minutes, turning halfway. Serve hot with healthy fries, dips and sauces.

hummus sandwiches 3 ways

Hummus sandwiches are a staple in our home. I am sharing with you three different styles of hummus sandwiches. I love all three sandwiches, but if I had to pick my favourite it would be the Mediterranean one. Feel free to swap ingredients around and use whatever you have in the fridge. My recipes are here to be used as a guide. You can use gluten-free bread, sourdough or wholemeal/whole-wheat seeded bread like I did. I used my homemade Oil-free Hummus recipe (see page 100) for these sandwiches.

HUMMUS, SULTANA & CARROT

1–2 slices wholemeal/whole-wheat seeded bread

1 tablespoon hummus (see page 100)

½ medium-sized carrot, grated or cut into thin ribbons

½ tablespoon sultanas

½ teaspoon ground cumin

MEDITERRANEAN HUMMUS

1–2 slices wholemeal/whole-wheat seeded bread

1 tablespoon hummus (see page 100)

4 sun-dried tomatoes halves

½ teaspoon dried Italian herbs

4 basil leaves (optional)

AVOCADO HUMMUS

1–2 slices wholemeal/whole-wheat seeded bread

1 tablespoon hummus (see page 100)

flesh from ½ avocado, sliced

¼ cucumber, sliced

½ teaspoon za'atar or ground cumin

EACH SANDWICH SERVES 1

PREP TIME: 10 MINUTES

Spread the hummus on one side of the bread then top with your chosen toppings and close the sandwich with the second slice of bread (if using) or serve as open sandwiches.

Serve or store in an airtight container in the fridge.

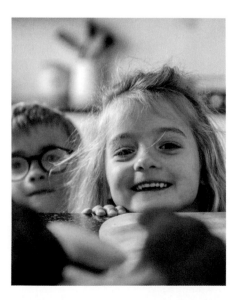

DF EF NF OF SF SYF

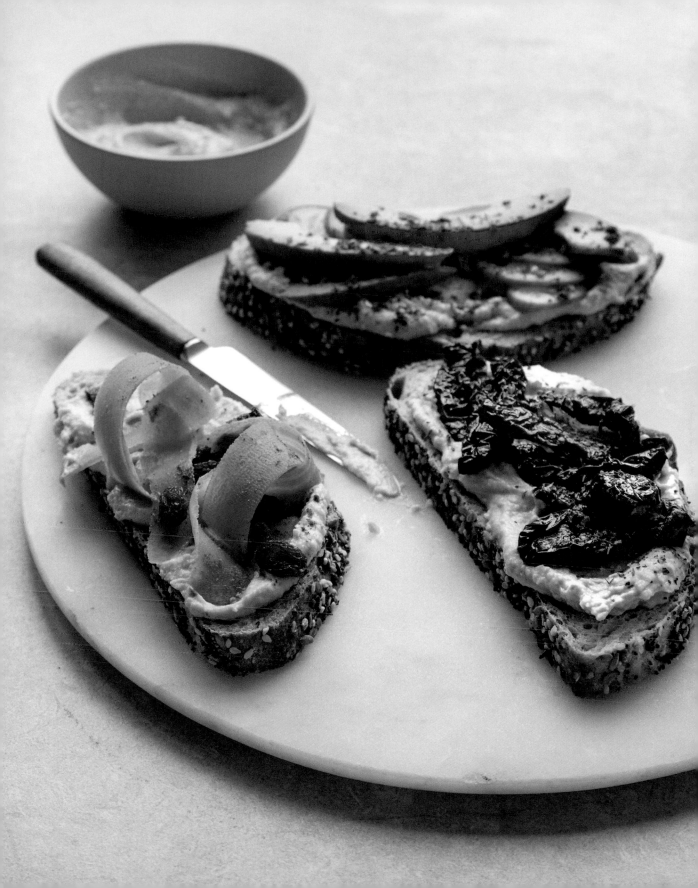

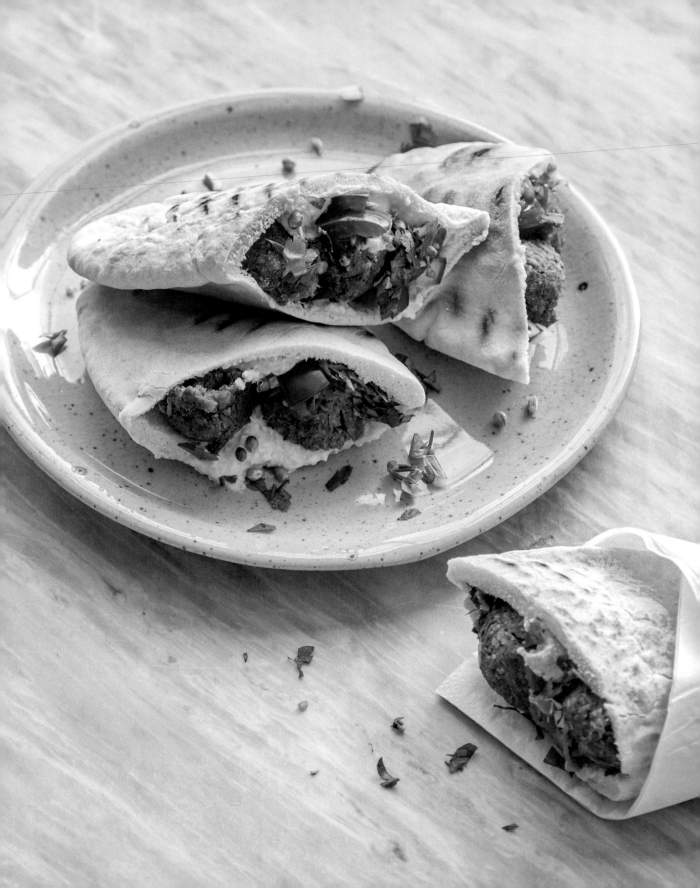

pitta sandwiches

We love love love Lebanese food in my family and these pitta sandwiches are on the menu every week for lunch! If you don't want to make the lentil bites, you could use pre-made falafels or canned chickpeas as a filling for convenience. I also like adding hemp seeds in my tabbouleh for extra plant-based nutrition. Feel free to add any veggies you like – the more the merrier! We usually have half a pitta bread each but eat more if you are extra hungry!

2 pitta breads
2 tablespoons hummus (see page 100)
8–10 Lentil Bites (see page 36), pre-made falafels or canned chickpeas, as preferred

TOMATO TABBOULEH
2 tomatoes, finely chopped
½ red onion, finely chopped
15 g/½ cup freshly chopped parsley
2 tablespoons hemp seeds
juice of ½ lemon
salt and pepper

SERVES 2–4

PREP TIME: 10 MINUTES
COOKING TIME: 2–3 MINUTES
(PLUS AN ADDITIONAL 25–30 MINUTES IF MAKING THE LENTIL BITES)

To make the tabbouleh, combine the tomatoes, red onion and parsley with the hemp seeds, lemon juice and salt and pepper.

Gently heat the pitta breads in a frying pan/skillet or sandwich-maker for 1–2 minutes each side, then slice in half widthways, or across, and open slightly to use as a pocket.

Spread the hummus inside the pitta pockets, add the lentil bites, if liked, and tomato tabbouleh then serve.

chickpea 'omelettes'

We love eating these chickpea 'omelettes' or crèpes for lunch filled with vegetables, mushrooms, baby spinach or vegan cheese. They are really nutritious and packed with plant-based protein. They are really convenient to make and also really easy. My little ones love them. Chickpea flour can be found in Indian grocers or most supermarkets and health food shops under the name gram, besan, or garbanzo bean flour.

80 g/⅔ cup chickpea flour
2 tablespoons nutritional yeast
pinch of ground turmeric
pinch of salt
50 g/1 cup cooked chopped chard
75 g/1 cup sautéed sliced
  mushrooms
olive oil, for frying

SERVES 2

PREP TIME: 2–5 MINUTES
COOKING TIME: 5 MINUTES

In a small bowl, whisk together the flour, nutritional yeast and turmeric with 180 ml/⅔ cup water until all the lumps are gone.

Heat a small frying pan/skillet over a medium heat and grease with olive oil.

Pour half of the batter evenly into the pan and cook over a medium heat for a few minutes before flipping it and cooking the other side for a few minutes.

Add the chopped chard and sauteed mushrooms before folding the pancake in half and transferring to a plate.

Cook the second omelette following the same method.

Variations: Add any of the following: ground cumin, crushed garlic, vegan cheese, diced avocado and your choice of vegetables and greens.

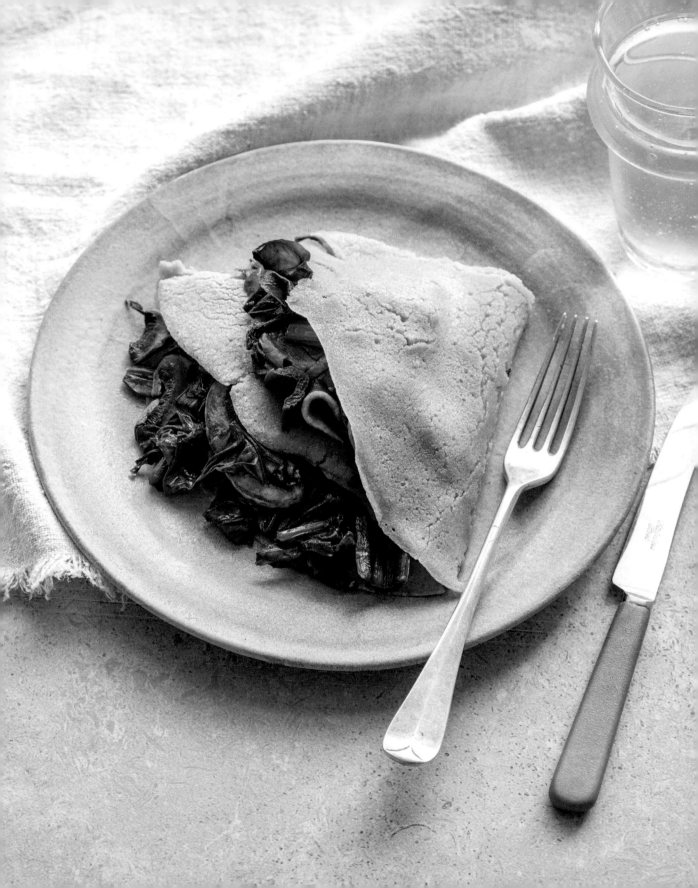

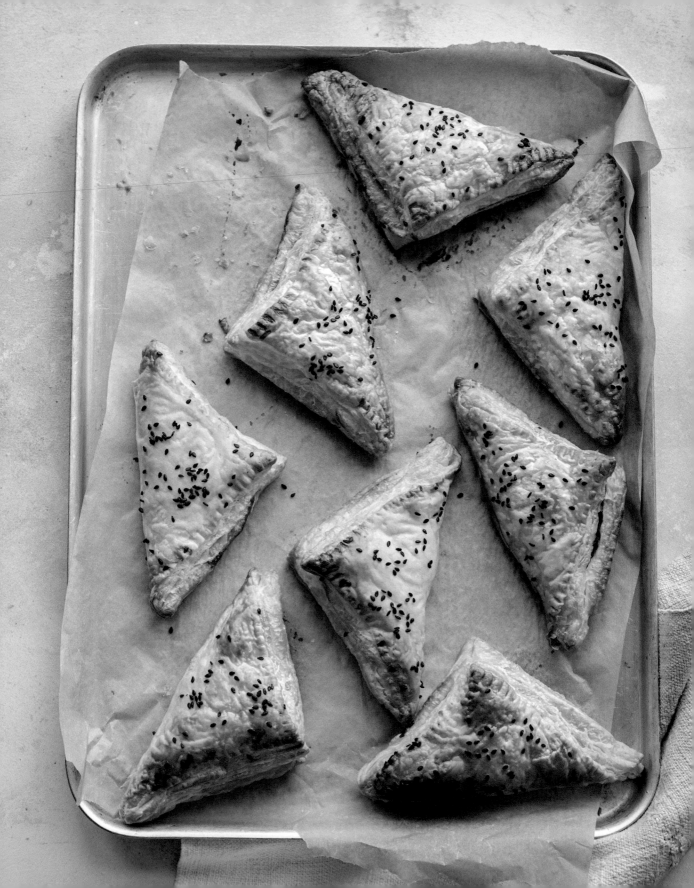

spinach & cashew 'ricotta' triangles

If you're looking for a delicious lunch or side dish to make for a BBQ party this is it. You could also use different fillings such as sun-dried tomatoes, vegan cheese or my pumpkin lentil 'sausage' roll mix. I used vegan puff pastry found in my local supermarket, but make sure to check the label before buying.

5 sheets frozen vegan puff pastry
150 g/1 cup raw cashews (soaked in cold water for 3–6 hours or in boiling water for 10 minutes), drained and rinsed
3 tablespoons nutritional yeast
1 teaspoon garlic powder
½ teaspoon onion powder
½ teaspoon sea salt
250 g/2 cups spinach
1 tablespoon soya milk
2 tablespoons black sesame seeds

2 x baking sheets lined with parchment paper

MAKES ABOUT 20

PREP TIME: 15 MINUTES
COOKING TIME: 40 MINUTES

Preheat the oven to 200°C (400°F) Gas 6.

Defrost the pastry sheets.

To make the filling, in a high-speed blender, blend the cashews together with 125 ml/½ cup cold water, the nutritional yeast, garlic powder, onion powder and sea salt until smooth and creamy.

Mix the spinach with the cashew cream and set aside.

Cut the pastry sheets into equal-sized squares (usually into four) then place 1 large tablespoon of the filling in the centre of each and fold each square into a triangle. Press down the two open sides with a fork to close gently and place them on the prepared baking sheet.

Using a pastry brush, gently brush each triangle with a little soya milk, then sprinkle some sesame seeds on top.

Bake them in the preheated oven for 20–25 minutes until golden brown. Remove from the oven and serve warm or cold.

DF EF
SF

pesto wholemeal scrolls

These make the best portable lunch option for kids' lunchboxes or picnics. I also like to make them for share plates or lunch with a salad. I like the pesto flavour the best, but you can also make them mini pizza scrolls. You can also use vegan puff pastry when short on time.

WHOLEMEAL DOUGH
180 ml/⅔ cup warm water
1 teaspoon active dried yeast
    granules
pinch of coconut sugar
300 g/2 cups wholemeal/
    whole-wheat flour, plus
    extra for dusting
pinch of sea salt
½ teaspoon dried Italian
    herbs
2 tablespoons olive oil

PESTO
1 bunch basil leaves
60 ml/¼ cup olive oil
30 g/¼ cup pine nuts
2 tablespoons nutritional yeast
pinch of sea salt

ovenproof baking dish, *lightly greased*

MAKES 10–12

PREP TIME: 1–2 HOURS
COOK TIME: 30–40 MINUTES

 DF EF
 SYF

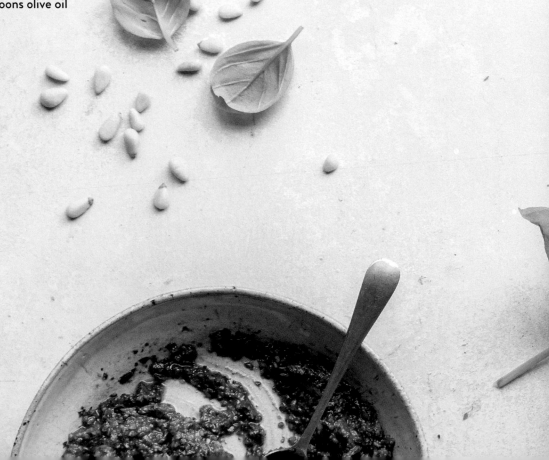

In a small bowl, combine the warm water, yeast and sugar, and stir until the yeast is dissolved. Let the water sit for about 5 minutes or until the yeast has activated and it starts to create bubbles in the water.

In a large mixing bowl, combine the flour with the salt and dried herbs.

Pour the olive oil into the yeast mixture and then pour it into the flour.

Stir to combine the flour with the water until it forms a large ball of dough. Then knead the dough on a clean surface dusted with flour. If too sticky, add a little extra flour. Knead the dough with your hands for about 5 minutes.

Put the dough back in the bowl, cover it with a kitchen towel and leave it to rise for about an hour at room temperature. Once it has risen, preheat the oven to 200°C (400°F) Gas 6.

Meanwhile, make the pesto by blending all the ingredients together in a blender or food processor to make a paste.

Remove the dough from the bowl and stretch the dough on a sheet of parchment paper to form a large rectangle, aiming to keep the dough nice and thin.

Once shaped, spread the pesto over the surface of the dough from edge to edge. Then slice into 2–3-cm/¾–1¼-inch wide strips using a knife and roll up each pesto scroll individually.

Put the sliced rolls into the prepared baking dish in a single layer. Make sure to use a dish large enough to allow the rolls room to expand as they bake. Bake in the preheated oven for about 30 minutes.

Serve warm or cold. Once cool, store them in an airtight container in the fridge.

Variations: Swap pesto for tomato purée/paste, vegan cheese and chopped spinach and olives or use vegan puff pastry instead of dough.

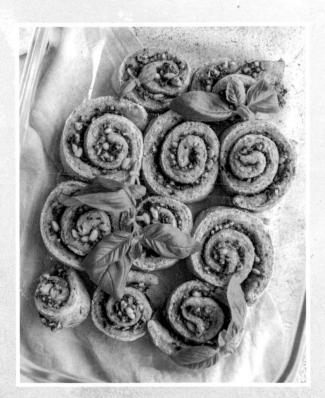

Mexican food really is the best for creating delicious plant-based meals. I try to pack a lot of healthy vegetables in our burritos as well as creamy guacamole and tasty rice and beans for a serving of plant protein. I roll the burritos in parchment paper to serve them like they do in Mexican restaurants, which helps the younger children to eat them without too much mess!

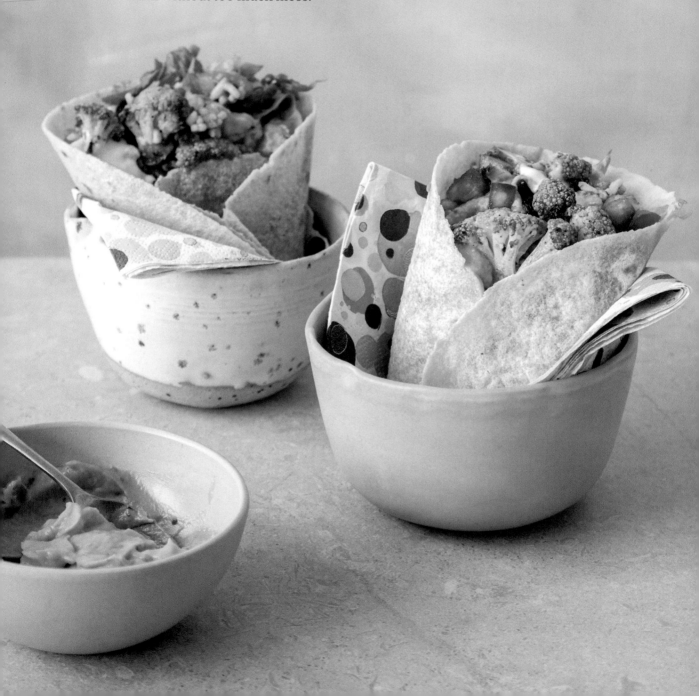

cauliflower burritos

1 small cauliflower or ½ medium
  cauliflower
1–2 teaspoons paprika
1 teaspoon onion powder
1 teaspoon garlic powder
500 g/2 cups cooked rice or
  200 g/1 cup uncooked rice
250 ml/1 cup tomato salsa
1 x 420-g//5-oz. can pinto or red
  kidney beans
guacamole
4 large corn tortillas
50 g/1 cup chopped lettuce
2–3 tomatoes, chopped
60 ml/¼ cup vegan sour cream
  or coconut yogurt
grated vegan cheese (optional)
salt and pepper

*baking sheet lined with parchment
  paper*

SERVES 4

PREP TIME: 15 MINUTES
COOKING TIME: 40 MINUTES

Preheat the oven to 200°C (400°F) Gas 6.

Cut the cauliflower into florets, season with the paprika and onion and garlic powders, spread out on the prepared baking sheet and bake in the preheated oven for 30 minutes.

Meanwhile, cook the rice (if needed) following the packet instructions.

Mix the cooked rice, salsa and beans together in a bowl.

To assemble the burritos, spread 1–2 tablespoons of guacamole onto the tortillas, then add a quarter of the rice mixture, a quarter of the baked cauliflower broken into small pieces, salt, pepper, lettuce, tomatoes and vegan sour cream or coconut yogurt and vegan cheese (if using).

Fold the bottom of the tortillas then fold the sides and serve.

Optional: Add in corn and/or cooked vegetables such as courgette/zucchini and red (bell) pepper/capsicum.

courgette chia meatless balls

These crunchy, tasty, meatless chia courgette/zucchini balls are really
good in pasta with a tomato sauce and spaghetti or with a nice salad.
I have also made them to pack for road trips as snacks.

1 large courgette/zucchini, grated
60 g/⅓ cup chia seeds
60 ml/¼ cup arrowroot powder
   or cornflour/cornstarch
60 ml/¼ cup olive oil
pinch of sea salt
1 teaspoon dried Italian herbs
½ teaspoon garlic powder
½ teaspoon onion powder
vegan hard cheese and basil leaves,
   to serve

*baking sheet lined with parchment
   paper*

MAKES 15

PREP TIME: 5–10 MINUTES
COOKING TIME: 20–25 MINUTES

Preheat the oven to 200°C (400°F) Gas 6.

Combine the grated courgette/zucchini in a mixing bowl
with the chia seeds, arrowroot or cornflour/cornstarch,
olive oil, salt, herbs and garlic and onion powders.
Combine well and add extra olive oil or arrowroot if the
mixture is too dry or too wet.

Roll the mixture into 15 even-size balls with your hands
and place them on the prepared baking sheet.

Bake in the preheated oven for 20–25 minutes, flipping
them over halfway through.

Serving suggestion: Serve hot with cooked pasta and
tomato sauce.

DF EF GF WF
NF SF SYF

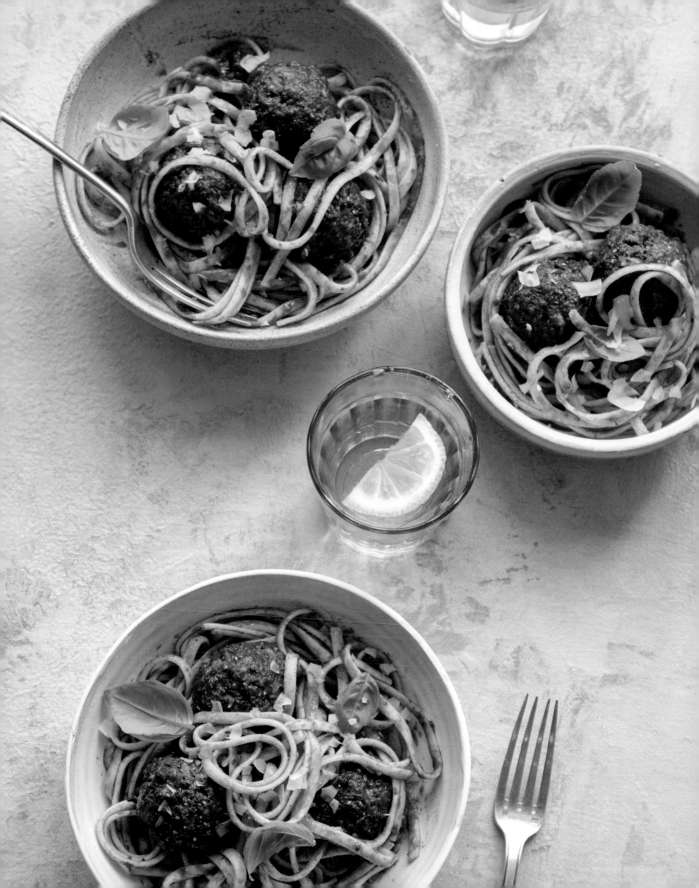

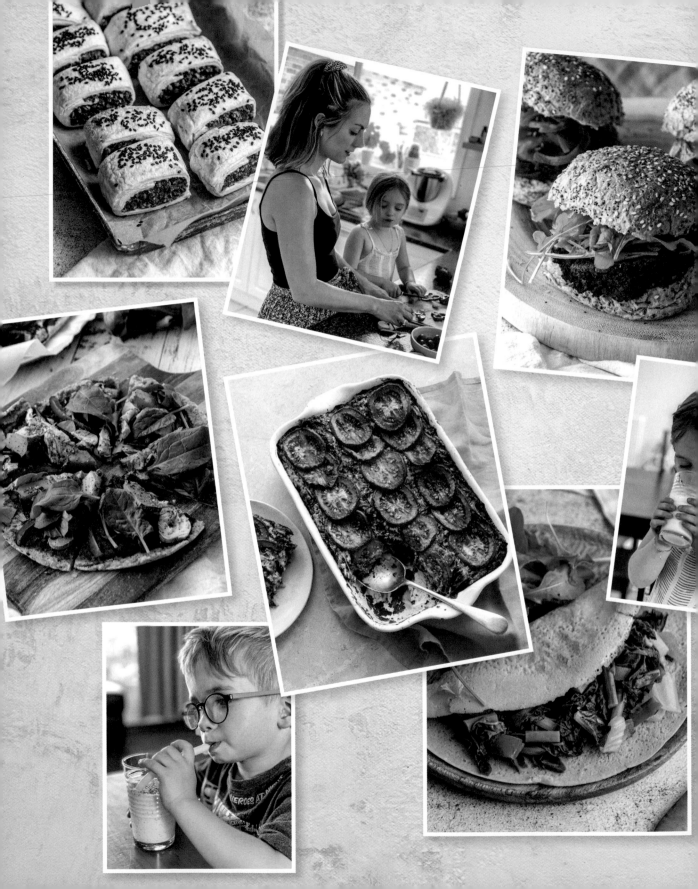

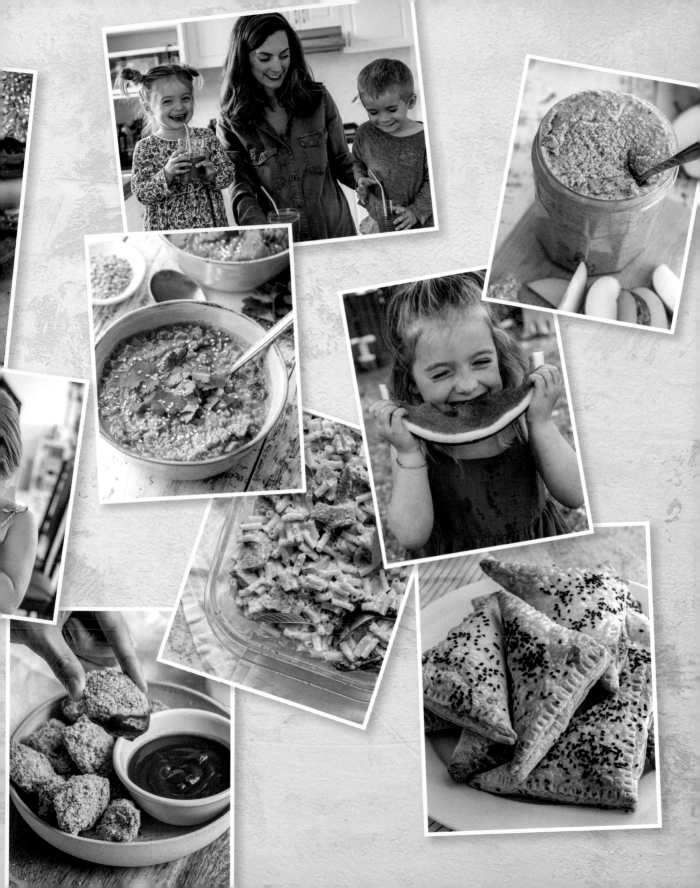

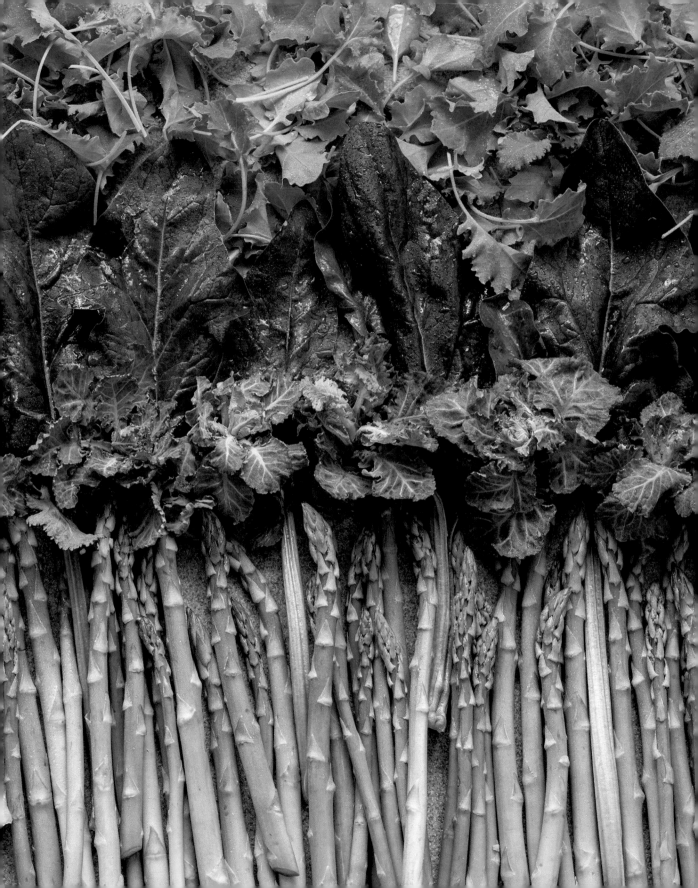

DINNER

tofu quinoa 'fried rice'

veggie nachos

spinach & cashew 'cheese' quesadillas

burgers 3 ways

baked fries & 2 dips

chickpea ratatouille stew

spinach & cashew 'ricotta' lasagne

cashew, squash & sage macaroni pasta bake

black bean tacos

creamy avocado pasta

quinoa mushroom risotto

broccoli pesto pasta

creamy mushroom & cashew pasta

rainbow spinach pizzas

red lentil pizza crusts

cauliflower potato cashew bake

vegetable pasta 'pistou' soup

sweet potato & red lentil soup

lentil dhal

pilau rice

chickpea satay curry

tofu quinoa 'fried rice'

My little family loves this healthy take on fried rice. With tofu for protein, quinoa for complex carbohydrates and quite a few veggies, it is a really simple but still healthy and delicious mid-week dinner that your family will love. You can swap quinoa for brown rice or swap the tofu for edamame beans. You can top them with spring onions/scallions, chilli/chili sauce, toasted nuts or sesame seeds. Also, I recommend soaking quinoa in cold water for a few hours before use.

180 g/1 cup quinoa (soaked for a few hours and rinsed)
1 tablespoon sesame oil
1–2-cm/½–¾-inch piece of fresh root ginger, peeled and finely diced
1 garlic clove, finely diced
1 onion, finely diced
2 carrots, finely diced
1 head broccoli, cut into small florets
75 g/½ cup frozen green peas
1 x 300-g/10½ oz. packet firm tofu
½ teaspoon ground turmeric
2 spring onions/scallions, chopped
2 teaspoons chilli/chili sauce/Sriracha (optional)
2 teaspoons sesame seeds, toasted (optional)
2 tablespoons tamari

SERVES 4

PREP TIME: 10 MINUTES
COOKING TIME: 20–25 MINUTES

Bring a saucepan of water to the boil. Add the soaked and rinsed quinoa and cook it until tender.

Meanwhile, heat the sesame oil in a large pan and add in the finely diced ginger, garlic and onion and cook for a few minutes until translucent.

Add in the diced carrots, broccoli florets and frozen green peas and cook with the lid on for 5–10 minutes until the carrots and broccoli are soft and cooked, stirring often with a spatula.

Add the firm tofu to the pan and break it up with the spatula. Add in the turmeric to give the tofu a more 'egg-like' look. Cook, stirring for a few minutes, then season with the tamari sauce.

Add the cooked quinoa to your pan and mix it with the tofu and veggies for a few minutes.

Serve in bowls and top with the spring onions/scallions. Add chilli/chili sauce and toasted sesame seeds, if desired.

Variations: Add edamame beans, swap the quinoa for brown rice, use red cabbage, Asian greens or pineapple.

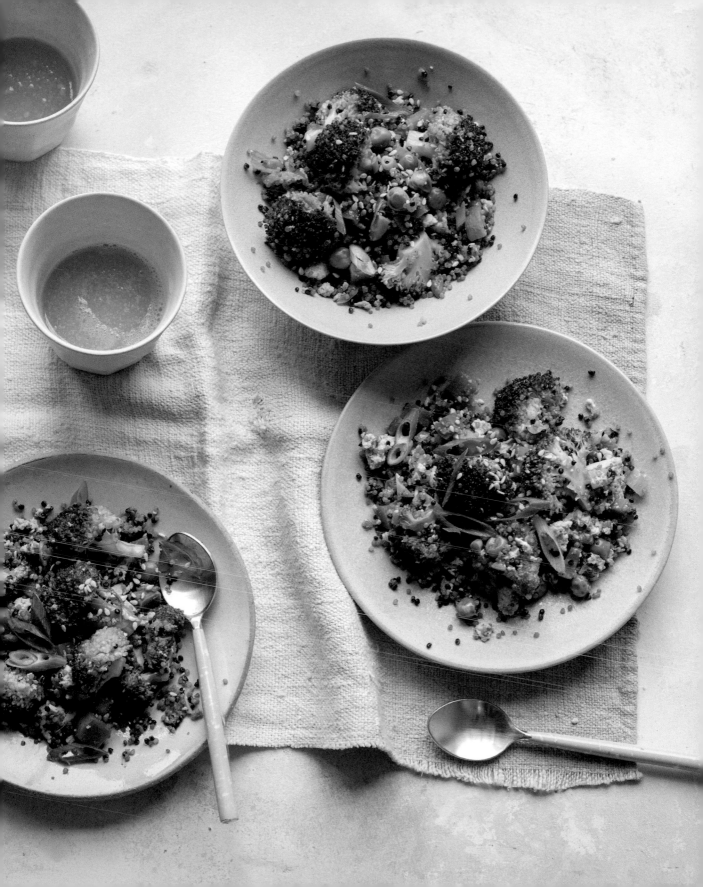

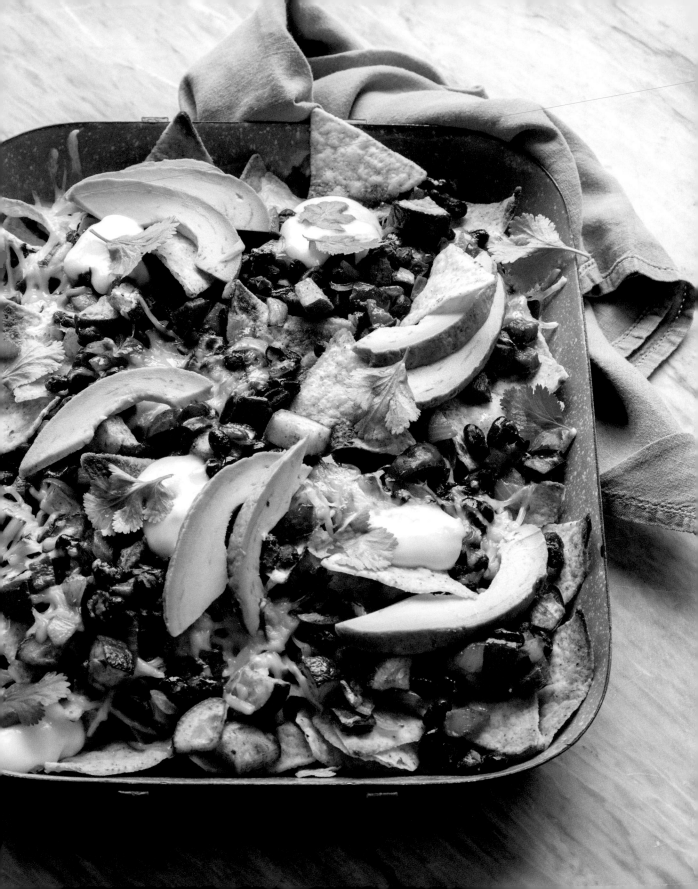

veggie nachos

Mexican dinners are a big hit in our family and I love how delicious and packed with veggies these nachos can be. I prefer using organic or natural corn tortilla chips. Feel free to swap some vegetables around depending on what you have in the fridge. Also, I keep my nachos not too hot and spicy and prefer adding jalapeños into the adults' plates to keep them mild and kid-friendly.

1 tablespoon olive oil
2 teaspoons paprika, plus extra for sprinkling
1 teaspoon ground cumin
1 teaspoon garlic powder
1 onion, diced
2 garlic cloves, crushed
2 small courgettes/zucchini, diced
1 red (bell) pepper/capsicum, diced
1 x 420-g/15-oz. can black beans
200 g/7 oz. corn tortilla chips
vegan hard cheese, grated
2–3 avocados, peeled, stoned and sliced (optional)
vegan sour cream (optional)
handful of jalapeños (optional)
handful of coriander/cilantro leaves (optional)

baking dish or baking sheet, lined with parchment paper

SERVES 4

PREP TIME: 10 MINUTES
COOKING TIME: 15–20 MINUTES

In a medium-sized pan, heat the olive oil and add in the spices to heat for a few seconds before adding the diced onion and garlic cloves and cooking them until translucent, stirring often with a wooden spatula.

Once the onion and garlic are cooked, add in the diced courgettes/zucchini and (bell) pepper/capsicum, cover and cook for 5 minutes, stirring often.

Drain and rinse the canned black beans and add to the spiced vegetables and stir to heat for a few minutes. Remove from the heat and set aside.

Preheat the grill/broiler to high. Spread the corn tortilla chips over the base of the prepared baking dish or baking sheet and top with the cooked vegetables. Sprinkle with more paprika, top with vegan cheese, if using, and grill/broil at 200°C (400°F) Gas 6 for 5 minutes or until the cheese is melted.

Serve in bowls and top with sliced avocado, vegan sour cream, jalapeños and/or coriander/cilantro leaves, if desired.

Variation: Use red kidney beans, mushrooms and corn and top with salsa and guacamole.

spinach & cashew 'cheese' quesadillas

When I need a quick and easy dinner mid-week I rely on these spinach and cashew 'cheese' quesadillas for a yummy plant-based dinner. Adding red kidney beans or black beans also means you get a dose of plant-based protein. You could swap the homemade cashew cheese for store bought vegan cheese and add your favourite toppings to the quesadillas such as salsa, guacamole or different cooked vegetables.

CASHEW CHEESE
150 g/1 cup raw cashews
3 tablespoons nutritional yeast
30 g/¼ cup tapioca/arrowroot
 flour
½ teaspoon garlic powder
250 ml/1 cup filtered water

QUESADILLAS
8 corn tortillas
40 g/1 cup baby spinach, chopped
1 teaspoon paprika
200 g/½ cup canned drained red
 kidney beans
olive oil, for frying
optional extra vegetables: onion,
 red (bell) pepper/capsicum, corn
 and/or courgette/zucchini, chilli/
 chile
green salad, salsa and guacamole,
 to serve

SERVES 4

**PREP TIME: 10 MINUTES PLUS
SOAKING TIME
COOKING TIME: 40 MINUTES**

To make the cashew cheese, soak the cashews in cold water for 3–6 hours or for 10 minutes in boiling water.

Drain and rinse the soaked cashews and blend in a high-speed blender or food processor along with the nutritional yeast, tapioca/arrowroot flour, garlic powder and water. Blend until smooth, scraping the side of the blender or bowl if required.

Heat up the cashew cheese sauce in a pan over a medium heat stirring often with a wooden spoon to thicken it up.

For the quesadillas, spread a layer of the cashew cheese on top of one tortilla, top with chopped spinach, paprika and red kidney beans, extra cooked vegetables, sliced chilli/chile if using and then top with another tortilla. Or you could make half quesadillas and fold each tortilla in half to make it easier to flip.

Heat up a frying pan/skillet with a little olive oil, if using, and place your quesadilla, one at a time, to heat up for a few minutes on each side until golden and crispy on the bottom, reducing the heat if necessary to prevent burning the tortilla. Transfer the quesadilla to a chopping board, leave to cool for a minute and then slice into three triangles. Serve with a salad and some salsa and guacamole for dipping.

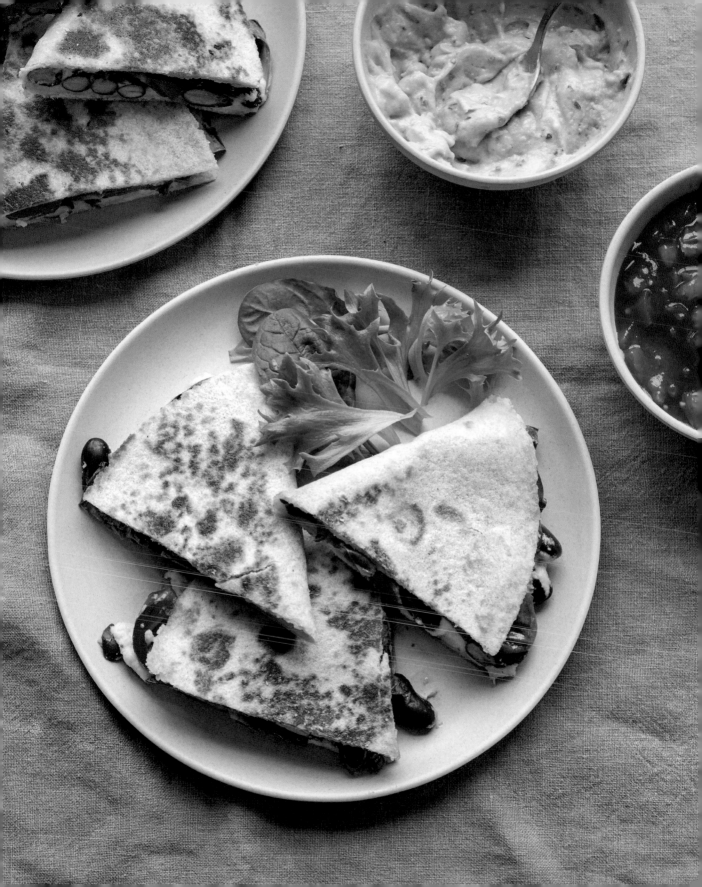

burgers 3 ways

Homemade burgers are a great satisfying dinner for the whole family. We switch between having mushroom burgers made with grilled/broiled Portobello mushrooms, homemade beetroot and black bean burgers or vegan 'beef' burgers with vegan cheese instead of the more traditional burger. Each recipe makes four burgers.

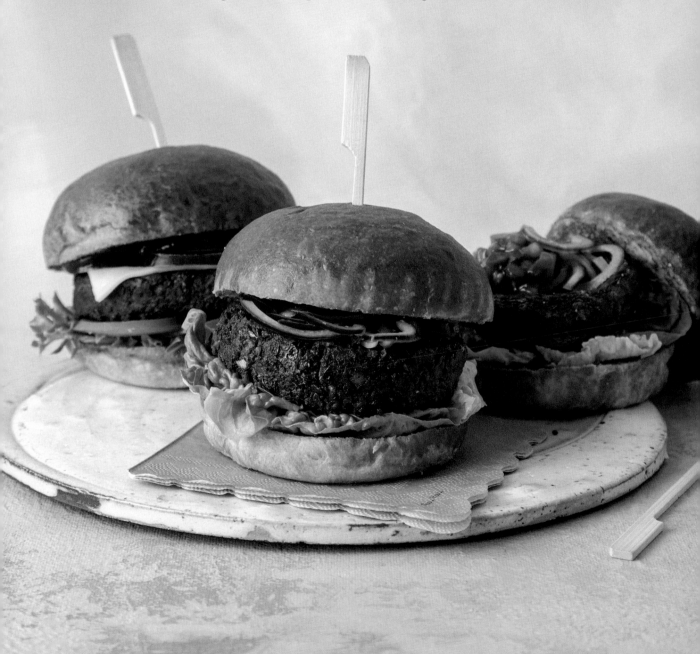

BEETROOT BEAN BURGERS

1 x 420-g/15-oz. can black beans,
    drained and rinsed
1 small beetroot/beet, peeled and
    diced
50 g/½ cup quick-cook oats
    or rolled oats
1 garlic clove, peeled and finely
    chopped
1 red onion, finely chopped
1 teaspoon curry powder
½ teaspoon sea salt
olive oil, for cooking

PORTOBELLO MUSHROOM BURGERS

4 Portobello mushrooms or large
    mushrooms
olive oil, for cooking

VEGAN CHEESEBURGERS

4 store-bought vegan 'beef'
    burgers
4 slices vegan Cheddar-style
    cheese
olive oil, for cooking

TO ASSEMBLE

4 teaspoons Dijon mustard
4 teaspoons vegan mayonnaise,
    tomato sauce or salsa
½ red onion or pickled onion,
    sliced
4 vegan burger buns, halved
1 tomato, sliced
4 lettuce leaves

EACH RECIPE MAKES 4 BURGERS

PREP TIME: 10 MINUTES
COOKING TIME: 20 MINUTES

To make the beetroot bean burgers, add the black beans to a food processor or blender and combine with all the remaining ingredients. Pulse a few times until all the ingredients are chopped finely and the mixture sticks together. Add extra oats if it is too wet.

Shape the burgers with your hands and place on a sheet of parchment paper on a tray or a plate and chill in the fridge for a few hours.

Cook the burgers in a pan with a little olive oil over a medium heat for 5 minutes on each side, flipping them very carefully. Remove from the heat.

FOR THE PORTOBELLO AND VEGAN BURGERS:
Cook the Portobello mushrooms or vegan burgers on the grill/BBQ or in a pan with a little olive oil.

TO ASSEMBLE ALL THE BURGERS:
Spread mustard, vegan mayonnaise or tomato sauce/salsa on the bun, then add the burgers and toppings.

Serve with a salad and enjoy.

baked fries & 2 dips

You don't have to give up your favourite foods to be healthy and plant-based, you just need to create healthier alternatives like these baked fries. I combine both sweet potatoes and white potatoes for even healthier fries. We like dipping them in homemade tomato sauce and a cheezy avocado dip. Served with a big salad and some beans, fries can be part of a healthy nutritious diet. I recommend soaking the cut-up potatoes in cold water for a few hours for extra crispy fries.

6 medium white potatoes
2 medium sweet potatoes
1 teaspoon dried herbs (optional)
sea salt, to serve

TOMATO SAUCE DIP
3 tablespoons tomato purée/paste
1 tablespoon maple syrup
2 teaspoons apple cider vinegar
½ teaspoon onion powder
pinch of sea salt

CHEEZY AVOCADO DIP
flesh from 2 ripe avocados
1 tablespoon nutritional yeast
1 tablespoon hemp seeds
freshly squeezed juice of 1 lemon
pinch of sea salt

*2–3 baking sheets, lined with
   parchment paper*

SERVES 2-4

**PREP TIME: 20 MINUTES PLUS 3-4
HOURS SOAKING TIME
COOKING TIME: 20-25 MINUTES**

Peel and slice the potatoes lengthways into fries. Put into a bowl, cover completely with cold water and leave to soak in the fridge for 3–4 hours.

Preheat the oven to 200°C (400°F) Gas 6.

Drain and rinse the potatoes and pat dry with a kitchen towel.

Lay the fries on the prepared baking sheets making sure they do not touch. Sprinkle them with herbs (optional).

Place the fries in the preheated oven and cook for 20–25 minutes until cooked and crispy.

While waiting for the fries to bake, make the dips. For each dip, mix the ingredients together in a bowl with a fork. Transfer to a small serving bowl, for dipping.

Serve the baked fries sprinkled with a little sea salt with dips and a salad.

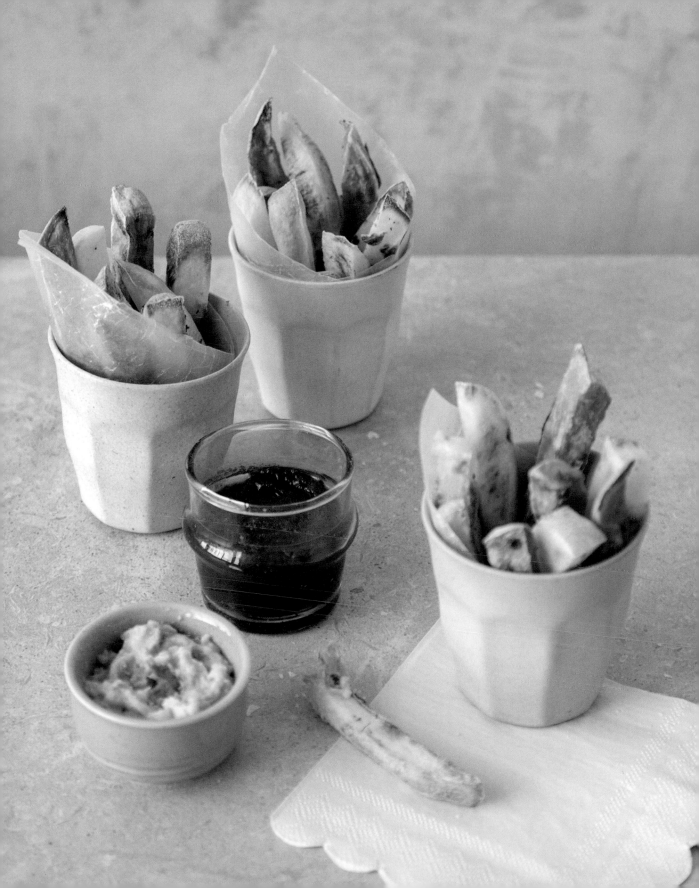

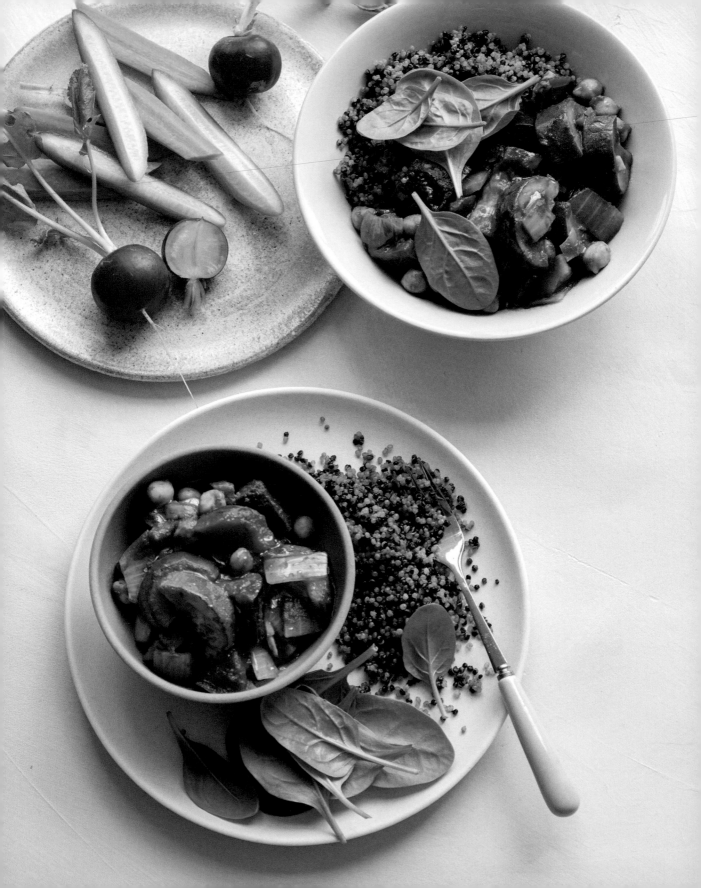

chickpea ratatouille stew

Being French, I grew up eating ratatouille. My version is a little bit
quicker to make (following my mum's recipe) and I added chickpeas for
an extra serving of legumes to make it a healthy, nutritious plant-based
dinner. I serve my stew with cooked quinoa, couscous or brown rice.

3 garlic cloves, crushed
1 onion, diced
1 tablespoon olive oil
1 teaspoon dried Italian herbs
quinoa or brown rice, to serve
1 large courgette/zucchini, sliced
1 red (bell) pepper/capsicum,
    deseeded and diced
1 aubergine/eggplant, diced
1 x 400-g/14-oz. can chopped
    tomatoes or same weight of
    fresh diced tomatoes or passata/
    strained tomatoes
1 x 400-g/14-oz. can chickpeas,
    drained and rinsed
salt and pepper
baby spinach and basil leaves,
    to serve (optional)

SERVES 4

PREP TIME: 15 MINUTES
COOKING TIME: 20–30 MINUTES

In a large pot over a medium heat, cook the garlic and
onion in the olive oil (or water if cooking oil-free) along
with the dried herbs. Cook for 5 minutes, stirring often,
until the onion is soft and translucent.

Meanwhile, cook the quinoa or rice following the packet
instructions.

Add the vegetables and tomatoes or passata to the
onion and garlic. Stir to combine and then cook, covered
with a lid stirring often, for 10–20 minutes until the
vegetables are soft. Add the chickpeas and combine.

Season with salt and pepper. Serve alongside the quinoa
or rice, with baby spinach and basil (if using).

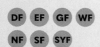

DF EF GF WF
NF SF SYF

cashew, squash & sage macaroni pasta bake

Every time I make this pasta bake my little boy eats two or three bowlfuls! I like to think my version with added greens and sage is adult-friendly and is fancy enough to share at dinner parties, too.

½ butternut squash, peeled, deseeded and diced
1 bunch of asparagus or 1 head of broccoli, diced
6–8 fresh sage leaves
150 g/1 cup raw cashews, soaked in cold water for 2–3 hours or for 10 minutes in boiling water
250 ml/1 cup cold water
15 g/¼ cup nutritional yeast
1 teaspoon onion powder
1 teaspoon garlic powder
500 g/18 oz. dried short-cut macaroni
salt and pepper

baking sheet lined with parchment paper
ovenproof casserole dish

SERVES 5–6

PREP TIME: 10 MINUTES
COOKING TIME: 35 MINUTES

Preheat the oven to 190°C (375°F) Gas 5.

Place the diced butternut squash and asparagus or broccoli onto the prepared baking sheet. Spread 5–6 sage leaves on top of the veggies. Cook them in the preheated oven for 25 minutes.

Meanwhile, make the cashew cheese sauce. Blend the drained and rinsed cashews, water, nutritional yeast, onion powder and garlic powder in a high-speed blender until smooth and creamy. Season with salt and pepper. Set aside.

In the meantime, cook the pasta following the packet instructions, then drain.

When the vegetables and pasta are cooked, combine the pasta, vegetables, sage leaves and cashew cheese sauce in an ovenproof casserole dish. Season with a little salt if required and top with sage leaves.

Put the pasta bake under a hot grill/broiler afor 10 minutes until golden. Remove from the oven and serve.

DF EF OF SF SYF

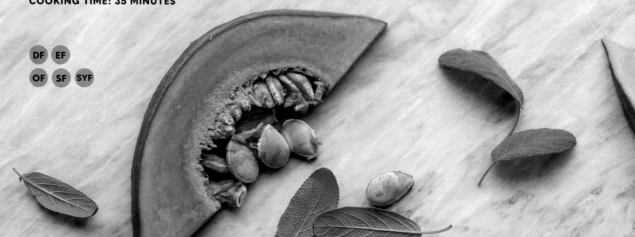

spinach & cashew 'ricotta' lasagne

This lasagne is really delicious and packed full of spinach. My kids love it so I hope yours do, too! You could make it gluten-free by using gluten-free lasagne sheets or layers of aubergine/eggplant instead.

150 g/1 cup raw cashews, soaked in cold water for 3 hours or for 10 minutes in boiling water
3 tablespoons nutritional yeast
1 teaspoon garlic powder
½ teaspoon onion powder
juice of ½ lemon
500 g/18 oz. baby spinach
700 g/25 oz. passata/strained tomatoes
250 g/9 oz. dried lasagne sheets
1 onion, diced
2 garlic cloves, crushed
2 tomatoes, sliced
salt and pepper, to season

ovenproof lasagne dish

SERVES 4–6

PREP TIME: 20 MINUTES
COOKING TIME: 45 MINUTES

Preheat the oven to 180°C (350°F) Gas 4.

Drain and rinse the cashews then blend in a high-speed blender with 160 ml/⅔ cup water, the nutritional yeast, garlic and onion powders, some salt and the lemon juice. Blend until smooth, then add the spinach and combine together. Set aside.

Assemble the lasagne. Pour a layer of passata/strained tomatoes into the base of the lasagne dish, add a layer of lasagne sheets, then some onion and garlic, more passata and lasagne sheets, then some of the spinach and cashew cheese and repeat again until the dish is full ending with a layer of spinach and cashew cheese. Top with sliced tomatoes and season with salt and pepper.

Bake in the preheated oven for 45 minutes. Remove from the oven and serve.

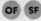

DF EF
OF SF SYF

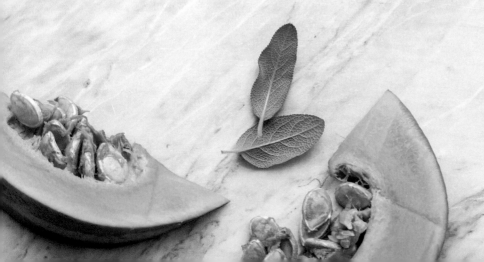

black bean tacos

Who doesn't love tacos?! Made with delicious vegetables, Mexican spices, black beans and wrapped in corn tortillas, they are my favourite homemade vegan tacos. I always end up putting too many toppings on and make a mess, but they are just so delicious! We love serving them with guacamole, coriander/cilantro, corn salsa or mango salsa, cashew cheese or vegan cheese and jalapeños to top.

2 garlic cloves, crushed
1 onion, diced
2 teaspoons paprika
1 teaspoon ground cumin
1 teaspoon garlic powder
1 teaspoon onion powder
1 red (bell) pepper/capsicum, deseeded and diced
1 courgette/zucchini, diced
1 x 420-g/15-oz. can black beans, drained and rinsed
kernels from 1 cob/ear corn
12 corn tortillas
olive oil, for cooking
salt and pepper, to taste
avocado, grated vegan cheese coriander/cilantro, jalapeños, mango salsa and lime wedges, to serve (optional)

TOMATO SALSA
3 tomatoes, finely diced
½ red onion, finely diced
handful of freshly chopped coriander/cilantro
juice of 1 lime

SERVES 4

PREP TIME: 5 MINUTES
COOKING TIME: 20 MINUTES

Heat a little olive oil, vegetable oil or water in a medium-sized pan over a medium heat. Add in the garlic and onion and stir for a few minutes, cooking until the onion is translucent. Add in all the spices and stir with the onion.

Add in the diced red (bell) pepper/capsicum and courgette/zucchini and cook with a lid on for 5 minutes, stirring often so as not to stick.

Add the black beans and corn kernels to the pan of vegetables for a few minutes to heat up. Season with salt and pepper.

While the veggies cook, make a tomato salsa (pico de gallo) by combining the finely diced tomatoes, red onion and coriander/cilantro in a bowl along with salt and pepper and the lime juice.

Heat the corn tortillas then fill with the black beans and vegetable mixture, tomato salsa and avocado or vegan cheese, coriander/cilantro and jalapeños, if you like.

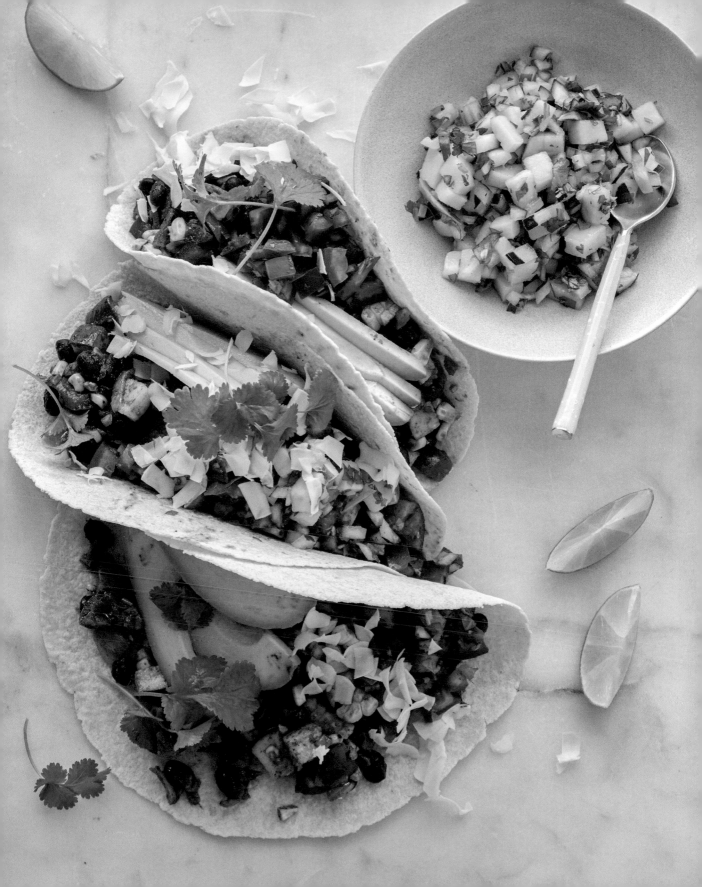

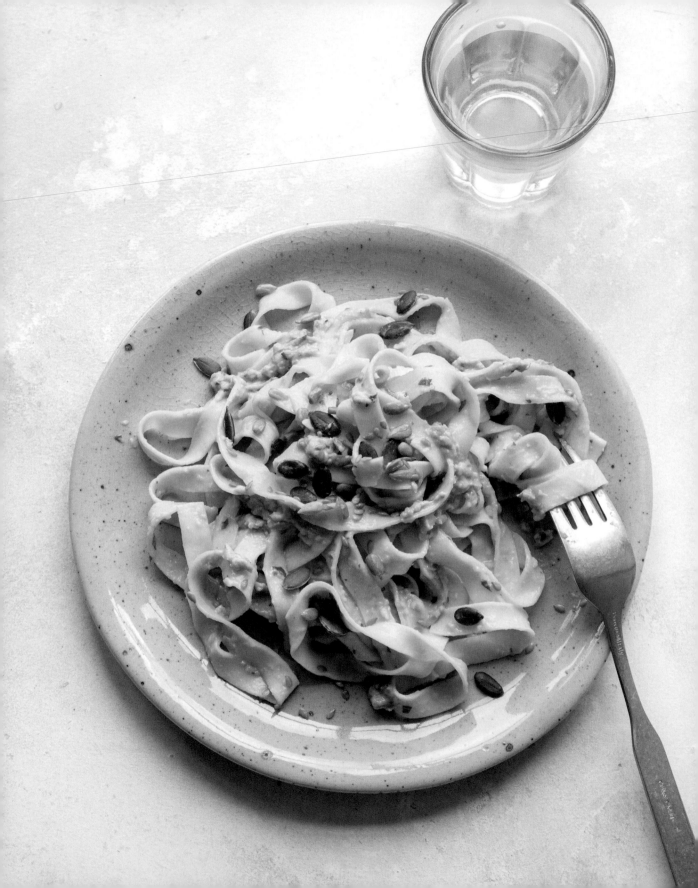

creamy avocado pasta

When I have a few ripe avocados, I love making this super-easy and delicious dinner. This pasta is also worth saving some avocados for. You cannot go wrong with a creamy avocado sauce and pasta! A big hit with kids, too! And with a little bit of fresh parsley, you increase your iron intake for the day! Win-win!

400 g/14 oz. dried pasta of choice
sunflower, pumpkin or mixed
   seeds of choice, to serve

CREAMY AVOCADO PASTA SAUCE
flesh from 4 small ripe avocados
15 g/¼ cup nutritional yeast
½ tablespoon olive oil
5 g/¼ cup freshly chopped parsley
1 garlic clove, peeled
½ teaspoon onion powder
1 tablespoon freshly squeezed
   lemon juice
salt and pepper, to taste

SERVES 4

PREP TIME: 5 MINUTES
COOKING TIME: 10–15 MINUTES

Cook the pasta following the packet instructions, then drain.

Put all of the pasta sauce ingredients into a blender, add 2 tablespoons cold water and blend for 1 minute or until the parsley and garlic are well blended in.

Pour the sauce into the cooked hot pasta, adjust the seasoning, toss to mix and transfer to serving plates. Top with seeds and serve.

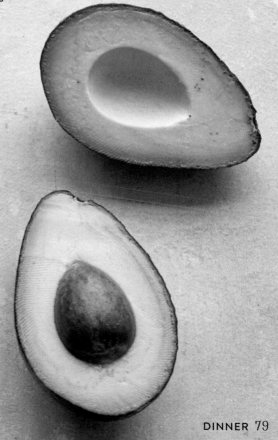

quinoa mushroom risotto

If you haven't tried quinoa risotto before, I recommend that you do.
I cook the quinoa the same way as I would Arborio rice for a risotto.
The end result is a delicious quinoa dish packed with flavour from the
mushrooms, herbs, garlic and lemon juice and the cheese taste is
achieved through nutritional yeast. This quinoa risotto could also be
made with pumpkin and sage or tomatoes and vegan sausages.

1 onion, diced
2 garlic cloves, crushed
1 tablespoon olive oil (optional)
1 teaspoon dried Italian herbs
1 x 500-g/18-oz. mushrooms,
　sliced
360 g/2 cups quinoa, rinsed
800 ml/3⅓ cups hot vegetable
　stock
juice of 1 lemon
20 g/⅓ cup nutritional yeast
handful of freshly chopped parsley
handful of freshly chopped thyme
sea salt and pepper
vegan Italian-style hard cheese
　shavings, to serve

SERVES 4

PREP TIME: 5-10 MINUTES
COOKING TIME: 30-40 MINUTES

Cook the onion and garlic in a large pan with the olive
oil (or water if cooking oil-free), stirring often. Add in
the dried Italian herbs and stir well.

Add the sliced mushrooms and cook over a medium
heat for a few minutes.

Once the mushrooms are cooked, combine the quinoa
with the mushrooms, onion and garlic and stir. Cover
the quinoa fully with some of the vegetable stock. When
the stock has been absorbed, add in the remaining
vegetable stock, a little at a time, on a high heat to let
the quinoa absorb the liquid, stirring regularly, until the
quinoa is soft and mushy.

Add some sea salt and pepper, the lemon juice,
nutritional yeast and some of the herbs and combine.

Top with vegan Italian-style cheese and the remaining
herbs and enjoy.

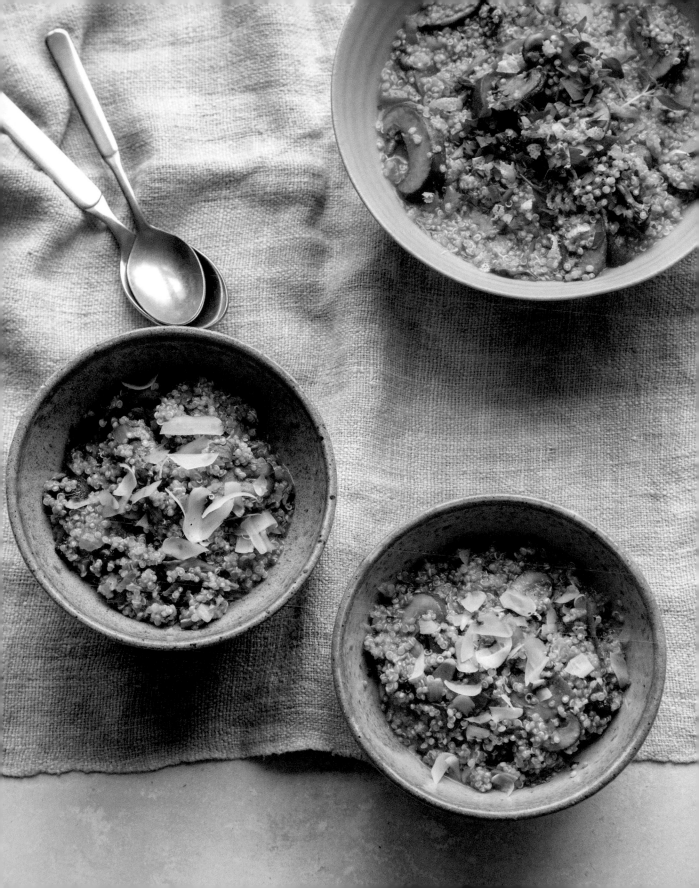

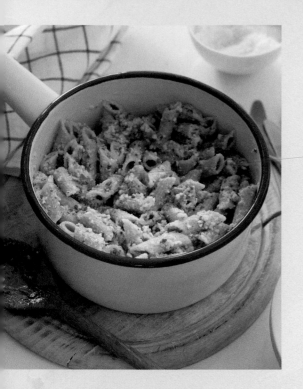

broccoli pesto pasta

Pasta is always a winner in our house, especially topped with this homemade broccoli pesto. We grow our own basil in summer and my twins love helping me water it, cut it and see me make the pesto. It makes this pasta even more delicious. Also, no one notices that I have hidden spinach and broccoli in the pesto so it is a mum win! This pesto is also delicious in toasted sandwiches, as a cold pasta salad dressing or with baked vegetables.

500 g/18 oz. dried pasta of choice

BROCCOLI PESTO
1 head broccoli
40 g/1 cup baby spinach
1 bunch of basil
10 g/¼ cup nutritional yeast
60 ml/¼ cup olive oil
60 ml/¼ cup water
1 garlic clove, peeled
juice of ½ lemon (optional)
salt and freshly ground black
    pepper, to taste

ADDITIONAL TOPPINGS
basil leaves
hemp seeds
nutritional yeast
vegan Italian-style hard cheese

SERVES 4–6

PREP TIME: 10 MINUTES
COOKING TIME: 10–15 MINUTES

Cook the pasta following the packet instructions, then drain.

In a high-speed blender, combine all of the broccoli pesto ingredients together and blend until smooth. Scrape the side of the blender if required. Season with salt and pepper.

Once the pasta is cooked, combine the pesto in the pot with the drained pasta. Stir to combine well and serve in bowls.

Top with extra basil, hemp seeds, nutritional yeast and/or vegan Italian-style hard cheese, as desired.

Store any leftover pesto in the fridge in an airtight container for up to 3 days.

DF EF
NF SF SYF

creamy mushroom & cashew pasta

I grew up on creamy mushroom pasta and I had to veganize the recipe my mum used to make us. I use the soaked cashews to make a creamy sauce and, combined with the mushrooms, wilted spinach and pine nuts, it is one of my favourite meals ever! And my kids' favourite, too!

500 g/18 oz. dried pasta of choice
1 onion, diced
1 garlic clove, crushed
500 g/2 cups mushrooms, diced
150 g/1 cup baby spinach
35 g/¼ cup pine nuts
olive oil, for cooking
salt and pepper

CASHEW CREAM
150 g/1 cup raw cashews soaked in cold water overnight or for 3–6 hours or for 10 minutes in boiling water
200 ml/¾ cup unsweetened almond milk
30 g/½ cup nutritional yeast
1 teaspoon onion powder
1 teaspoon garlic powder
½ teaspoon sea salt

SERVES 4–6

PREP TIME: 10 MINUTES
COOKING TIME: 15–20 MINUTES

Heat a little olive oil or water in a pan over a medium heat and cook the onion, garlic and mushrooms together, stirring often, until cooked.

While the mushrooms cook, make the cashew cream. Drain, rinse and blend the cashews in a high-speed blender with all of the remaining cashew cream ingredients until smooth and creamy.

Meanwhile, cook the pasta following the packet instructions, then drain.

Once the mushrooms are cooked, add in the baby spinach and stir in the cashew cream. Heat slowly over a low heat, stirring gently.

Combine the hot pasta and mushroom cashew cream together. Season with salt and pepper, and top with the pine nuts, then serve.

Variation: Add parsley, broccoli and peas.

rainbow spinach pizzas

This pizza is a hit with children and especially toddlers who love rainbows! It is also a great pizza to make with children to get them involved. As a nutritionist and mum I like the fact that the base has some extra spinach hiding! For the veggies, choose any vegetables in season to correspond with the colours of the rainbow. You can also add vegan cheese or keep it cheese-free.

SPINACH PIZZA DOUGH
30 ml/⅛ cup plus 1 tablespoon warm water
75 g/1 cup baby spinach
½ teaspoon coconut sugar
2 teaspoons active dried yeast granules
500 g/3½ cups pizza flour (type 00)
2 tablespoons olive oil
1 teaspoon sea salt

PIZZA TOPPINGS
125 ml/½ cup passata/strained tomatoes or tomato purée/paste
1 yellow, 1 orange and 1 green (bell) pepper/capsicum, deseeded and diced
1 red onion, diced
200 g/7 oz. cherry tomatoes, halved
1 teaspoon dried Italian herbs

2 pizza pans lined with parchment paper

MAKES 2 MEDIUM PIZZAS

PREP TIME: 20 MINUTES (PLUS 30–60 MINUTES FOR THE DOUGH TO RISE)

COOKING TIME: 25–30 MINUTES

In a blender combine the warm water and spinach and blend until finely chopped.

Pour the warm spinach water into a large bowl and add the coconut sugar and dried yeast. Whisk briefly to mix. Leave for a few minutes.

Add the flour, olive oil and salt to the bowl and combine with a spoon, then with your hands, to form a large ball of pizza dough. Cover with a kitchen towel and set aside in a warm place to rise for 30–60 minutes.

Preheat the oven to 200°C (400°F) Gas 6.

Knead the pizza dough for a few minutes until soft. Divide the dough in half and roll out two large, thin pizza bases. Try to get the bases as thin as possible. Place each base in a lined pizza pan. Spread a layer of passata/strained tomatoes or tomato purée/paste over the bases, then top each pizza with rainbow-coloured vegetables and bake them in the preheated oven for 25–30 minutes. Serve hot, cut into slices.

Other rainbow veggie ideas: red cabbage, red (bell) pepper/capsicum, carrot, corn kernels, squash, beetroot, spinach.

Optional: grated vegan cheese.

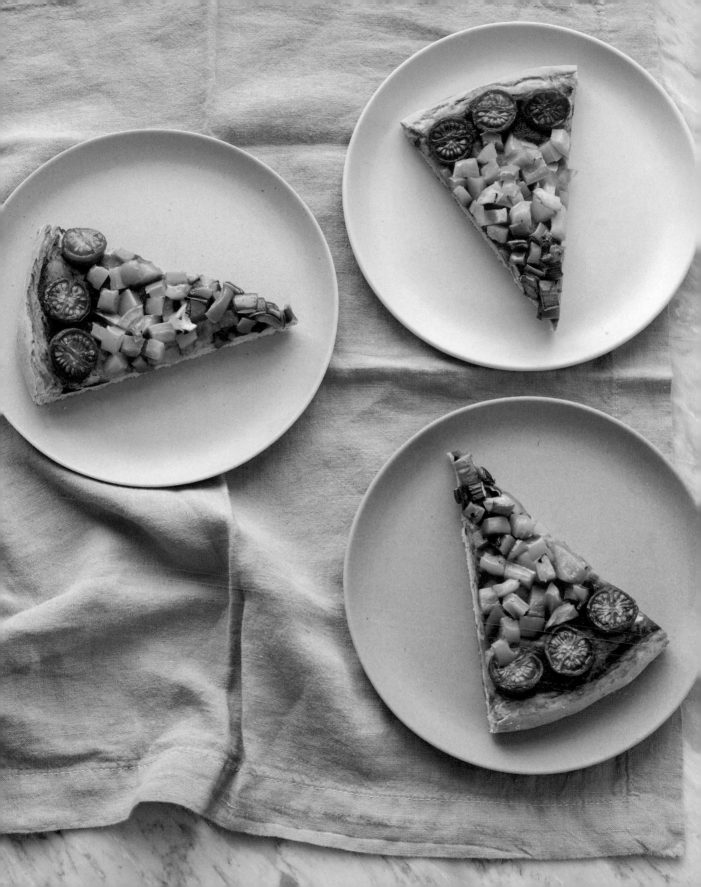

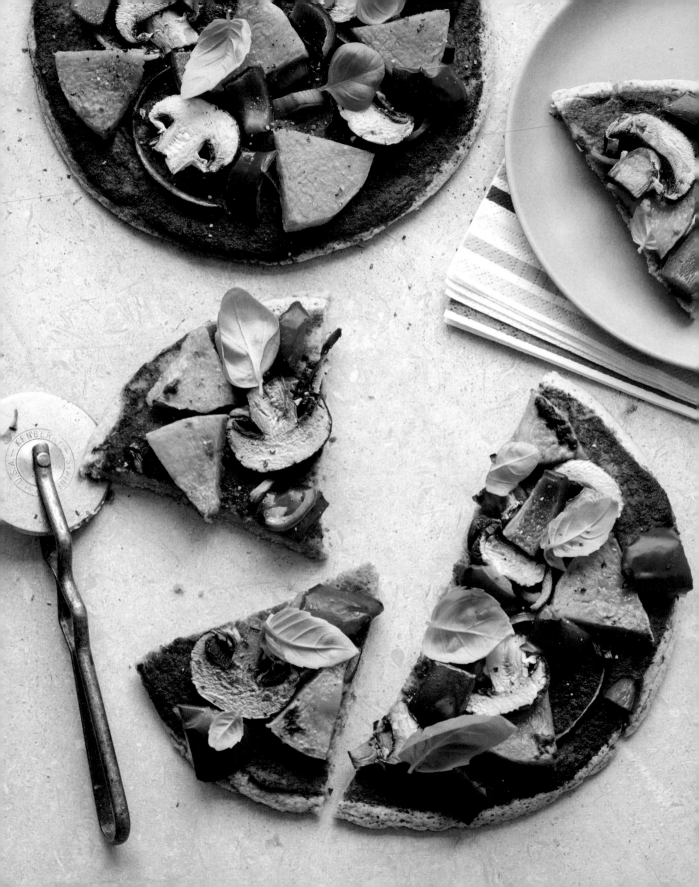

red lentil pizza crusts

Move over cauliflower crusts, I have a new healthy pizza crust recipe for you! It is actually very simple to make and includes uncooked red lentils to create a crusty pizza base high in vegan protein. Top with some passata, pizza paste and your favourite vegan pizza toppings!

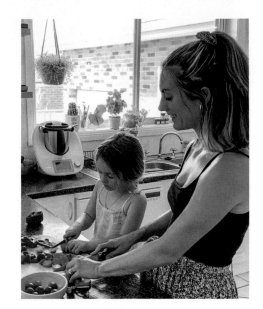

FOR THE PIZZA CRUSTS
400 g/2 cups dried red lentils
1 tablespoon dried Italian herbs
1 teaspoon garlic powder
1 teaspoon onion powder
olive oil spray

FOR THE TOPPING
4–5 tablespoons passata/strained
    tomatoes
½ red onion, thinly sliced
flesh from ⅓ roasted pumpkin
    or squash chopped
4–5 mushrooms, sliced
1 red (bell) pepper/capsicum,
    deseeded and chopped
handful of basil or spinach leaves
sea salt and freshly ground
    black pepper

MAKES 4 SMALL PIZZAS

PREP TIME: 5–10 MINUTES
COOKING TIME: 10–15 MINUTES

Rinse the dried red lentils and drain then blend in a food processor with the herbs and spices and 500 ml/2 cups cold water, until the lentils are broken down completely and the mixture is thick.

Spray a non-stick frying pan/skillet with a little olive oil spray, set over a medium heat and pour ¾ cup of the mixture into the pan spreading it out evenly. Cook for 3–4 minutes on one side before flipping and cooking for a further 1–2 minutes. Remove to a plate/board. Repeat with the other three crusts.

Place one pizza crust onto a baking sheet. Spread a generous tablespoon of passata/strained tomatoes over the crust and top with some of the vegetables. Put the pizza under a preheated grill/broiler and cook for 10–15 minutes.

Top with some basil or spinach leaves and season with salt and pepper. Remove to a plate to serve. Repeat for the remaining crusts.

Variation: Add grated vegan cheese and chopped pine nuts before grilling/broiling.

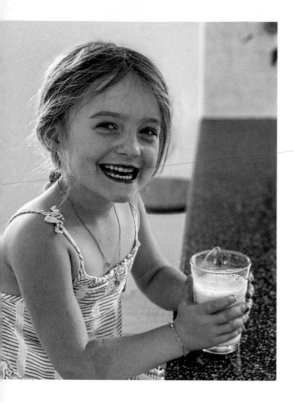

cauliflower potato cashew bake

I grew up eating cauliflower potato bakes on Sundays loaded with cream and cheese, but being vegan doesn't mean you have to miss out. I have recreated my mum's cauliflower potato bake with a cashew cream sauce and it is so delicious. Also a delicious way to eat cauliflower! This dish is a big crowd-pleaser!

Preheat the oven to 180°C (350°F) Gas 4.

Cook the potatoes and cauliflower in a pan of boiling water until al dente (approximately 20 minutes). Drain and transfer to an ovenproof baking dish.

Meanwhile, drain and rinse the soaked cashews and add them to a high-speed blender with 250 ml/1 cup water, the nutritional yeast, olive oil, spices and some salt and pepper. Blend until smooth and combined.

Pour the sauce over the potatoes and cauliflower in the baking dish.

Cover with foil and bake in the preheated oven for 45 minutes. Uncover and finish under a preheated grill/broiler until lightly browned on top. Serve.

Variation: Add broccoli or diced onions.

3–4 potatoes, peeled and diced
½ head cauliflower, cut into florets
150 g/1 cup raw cashews soaked in cold water for 2–3 hours or for 10 minutes in boiling water
2 tablespoons nutritional yeast
1 tablespoon olive oil
1 teaspoon paprika
1 teaspoon garlic powder
1 teaspoon onion powder
½ teaspoon grated nutmeg
½ teaspoon sea salt
½ teaspoon ground black pepper

oven-proof baking dish

SERVES 4–6

PREP TIME: 10–15 MINUTES
COOKING TIME: 1 HOUR

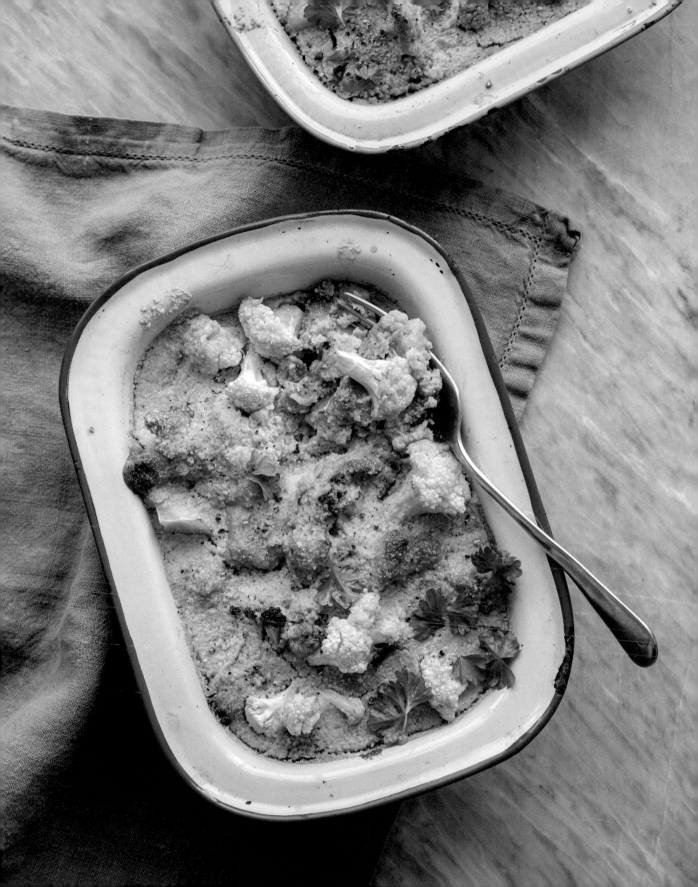

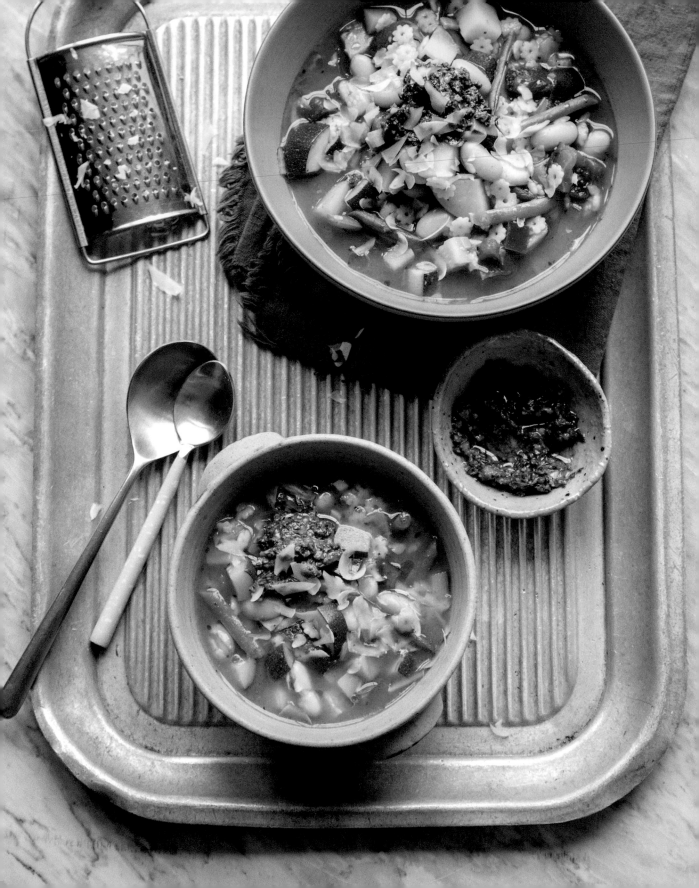

vegetable pasta 'pistou' soup

This soup is my vegan version of the vegetable pasta 'pistou' soup which comes from the South of France and uses pistou, which is similar to pesto. It is my son's favourite soup and it is a great nutritious meal for both winter and summer, full of fibre, protein and delicious basil. The traditional way of serving the soup is to add the pistou on top, but you can also combine it in the soup. I have also blended the soup in the past for picky eaters!

1 onion, diced
3 garlic cloves, crushed
1 tablespoon olive oil
125 g/1 cup green beans, chopped
2–3 small potatoes, diced
3 tomatoes, diced
2 courgettes/zucchini, diced
1 teaspoon dried Italian herbs
1 litre/4 cups vegetable stock
1 x 420-g/15-oz. can cannellini
   beans, drained and rinsed
70–100 g/2½–3½ oz. dried small
   pasta of choice
salt and pepper
vegan hard cheese, grated
   (optional), to serve

PISTOU/PESTO
1 bunch/1 cup basil leaves
2 garlic cloves, peeled
2 tablespoons pine nuts
2 tablespoons olive oil

SERVES 8

PREP TIME: 20 MINUTES
COOKING TIME: 40 MINUTES

Cook the onion and garlic in the olive oil in a large pot over a medium heat, stirring often.

Add the diced vegetables to the pot, stir well and add the dried Italian herbs. Pour in the vegetable stock, combine, increase the heat to high and bring to the boil.

Once boiling, reduce the heat to medium and cook for 5 minutes with a lid on.

Add the cannellini beans and dried pasta to the soup and stir to combine. Keep cooking on a medium heat covered with a lid for 20–30 minutes or until the potatoes and pasta are cooked. Season with salt and pepper.

Meanwhile, make the pistou sauce. In a blender or using a mortar and pestle, combine the basil, garlic cloves, pine nuts and olive oil to make a paste.

Serve the soup in bowls and add a dollop of pistou sauce to each bowl or stir it into the soup before serving. You can also blend the soup until smooth or simply serve it chunky as I do.

sweet potato & red lentil soup

We have a family tradition of making a fresh batch of soup every Sunday night. I love starting the week feeling nourished and healthy and it is so convenient having leftover soup for our Monday lunch! This sweet potato lentil soup is the family's favourite, hence why it is in my cookbook! Packed with protein from the lentils and complex carbohydrates from the sweet potatoes, it is nourishing, filling and makes us feel warm and healthy.

1 onion, diced
3 garlic cloves, crushed
½ tablespoon olive oil
3 tablespoons vegan Thai red curry paste or 1 tablespoon curry powder
300 g/1½ cups dried red lentils
2 large sweet potatoes, diced
1.5 litres/6 cups vegetable stock
1 x 400-g/14-oz. can chopped tomatoes
1 x 400-ml/14-fl oz. can coconut milk
salt and pepper

TO SERVE
handful of coriander/cilantro leaves
60 ml/¼ cup coconut yogurt

SERVES 4

PREP TIME: 10 MINUTES
COOKING TIME: 40 MINUTES

Cook the onion and garlic in a splash of water or the olive oil in a large pot for a few minutes until translucent, stirring often. Add the red curry paste or curry powder and stir to combine.

Rinse and drain the red lentils and add to the large pot along with the sweet potatoes and vegetable stock. Combine together and cover the pot.

Bring to the boil, then reduce the heat to medium and cook for 30 minutes, stirring often, until the lentils and sweet potatoes are soft.

Reduce the heat and add in the chopped tomatoes and coconut milk. Stir to combine and cook for a few minutes. Season with salt and pepper according to taste.

Serve in bowls with coriander/cilantro on top of each serving and a dollop of coconut yogurt.

Variations: add in extra vegetables, such as cauliflower, broccoli and peas and serve with crusty bread.

lentil dhal

This recipe is the one I always share with friends who want to try eating more plant-based meals. Eating this dish shows how good vegan dishes can be! And best of all this curry is so easy to make. Feel free to swap around the vegetables in it. I like adding lots of greens as it is a good way to add extra greens into our day.

2 teaspoons olive oil
1 teaspoon sea salt
½ teaspoon onion powder
½ teaspoon garlic powder
2 teaspoons curry powder
½ teaspoon ground ginger
½ teaspoon ground turmeric
½ teaspoon garam masala
½ teaspoon mustard powder
1 onion, diced
400 g/2 cups dried red lentils,
    rinsed and drained
1½ cups green vegetables (spinach,
    peas or diced courgette/
    zucchini, broccoli or cauliflower)
1 x 400-g/14-oz. can chopped
    tomatoes
1 x 400-g/14-oz. can coconut milk
cooked basmati rice, to serve
coconut yogurt, black pepper,
    coriander/cilantro, to serve

SERVES 6

PREP TIME: 5 MINUTES
COOKING TIME: 40–50 MINUTES

In a large pot, heat the olive oil over a medium heat and add the salt and all the flavourings and spices. Add the diced onion and cook until soft and translucent, stirring often.

Add in the rinsed and drained dried lentils along with 1 litre/4 cups water and combine.

Cover the pot with a lid, bring the water to the boil then reduce the heat to medium and add the vegetables.

Cook for 30–40 minutes or until the lentils are soft, stirring often.

Add in the tomatoes and coconut milk and stir to combine. Cook for 2–5 minutes more, then serve the dhal with cooked rice, a dollop of coconut yogurt, some black pepper and coriander/cilantro, if desired.

Variations: Add sliced chilli/chile, diced sweet potato, cauliflower, broccoli, carrot, courgette/zucchini green peas, spinach.

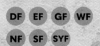

pilau rice

Whenever I cook rice I tend to cook too much and this dish is perfect to use up leftover rice. Packed with vegetables and flavour it is an ideal budget-friendly midweek dinner. I like ours with frozen green peas and broccoli but you could swap them for cauliflower, green beans or whatever vegetables you have to use up in your fridge. Top with coriander/cilantro and coconut yogurt.

2 teaspoons coconut oil
1 large onion, diced
3 garlic cloves, crushed
2 teaspoons mustard powder
2 teaspoons curry powder
1 teaspoon ground turmeric
1 teaspoon onion powder
75 g/½ cup frozen green peas
1 head broccoli, cut into florets
75 g/½ cup sultanas
75 g/½ cup raw cashews
500 g/2 cups cooked basmati rice
bunch of coriander/cilantro leaves
sea salt and pepper, to taste

TO SERVE
chilli/hot red pepper flakes
   (optional)
coconut yogurt (optional)

SERVES 4

PREP TIME: 10 MINUTES
COOKING TIME: 15 MINUTES

Heat the coconut oil in a large pan. Add the onion and garlic and cook, stirring often, until translucent. Add the spices, onion powder, frozen green peas and broccoli, cover and cook over a medium heat until soft.

Add the sultanas and cashews into the pan and combine briefly.

Pour the cooked rice into the pan and stir to combine the rice thoroughly. Season with salt and pepper. Heat up the rice in the pan for a few minutes until piping hot then serve into bowls and top with coriander/cilantro leaves and dried chilli/hot red pepper flakes and coconut yogurt, if desired.

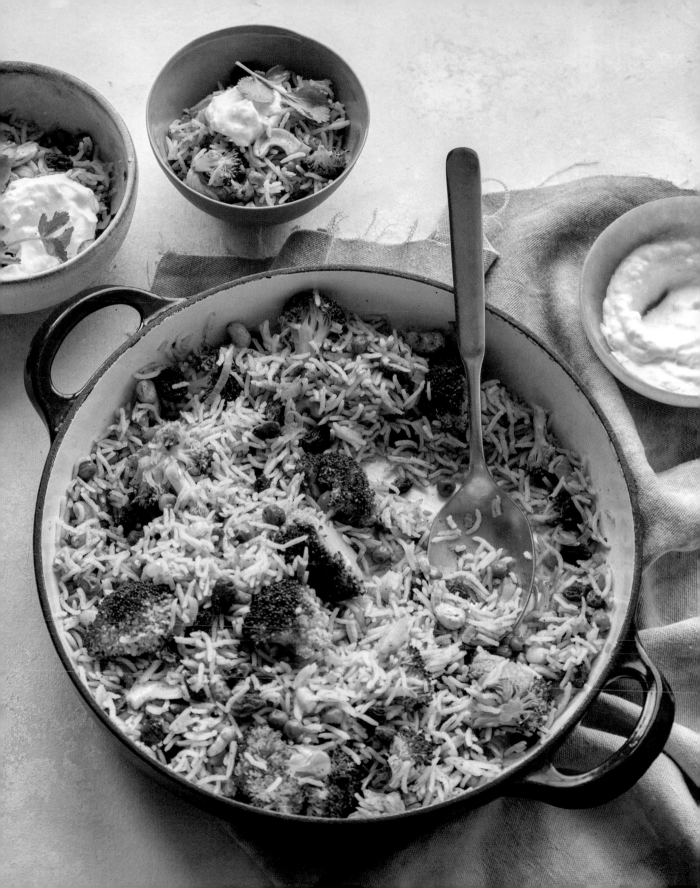

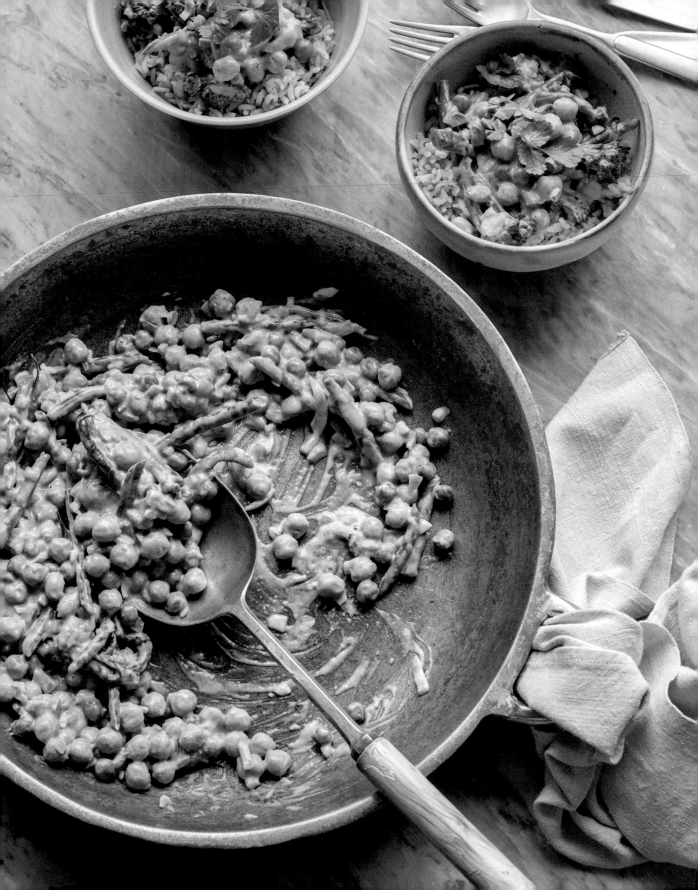

chickpea satay curry

Curry nights are my favourite nights of the week! We eat a lot of homemade vegan curries in our home and this chickpea satay is one of our favourites. It is very simple to make and is packed with plant protein and is really delicious and creamy with the peanut butter and coconut milk. You can use green beans, green peas, carrots, courgette/zucchini, broccoli or cauliflower for this dish. Serve with cooked basmati or brown rice.

2 garlic cloves, crushed
1 onion, diced
150 g/2 cups prepped vegetables (such as peas, beans and/or broccoli)
1 x 420-g/15-oz. can chickpeas, drained and rinsed
160 ml/⅔ cup coconut milk
1–2 tablespoons tamari sauce
125 g/½ cup peanut butter
juice of 1 lime
2 teaspoons sesame or peanut oil
basmati or brown rice, to serve
coriander/cilantro leaves, chopped peanuts, sliced chilli/chile, to serve (optional)

SERVES 4

PREP TIME: 5 MINUTES
COOKING TIME: 20 MINUTES

In a pan, heat the oil and cook the garlic and onion together for a few minutes.

Add in the green vegetables, stir to combine and cook on a low heat with the lid on until the vegetables are partly cooked. Add the chickpeas and stir.

For the sauce, combine the coconut milk with the tamari and peanut butter in a bowl and whisk to mix with a fork. Pour it into the curry and mix it with the vegetables.

Cook on a low heat for 5 minutes until heated through.

Squeeze over the lime juice and top with coriander/cilantro, peanuts and sliced chilli/chile to serve, if desired. Serve with cooked rice.

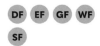

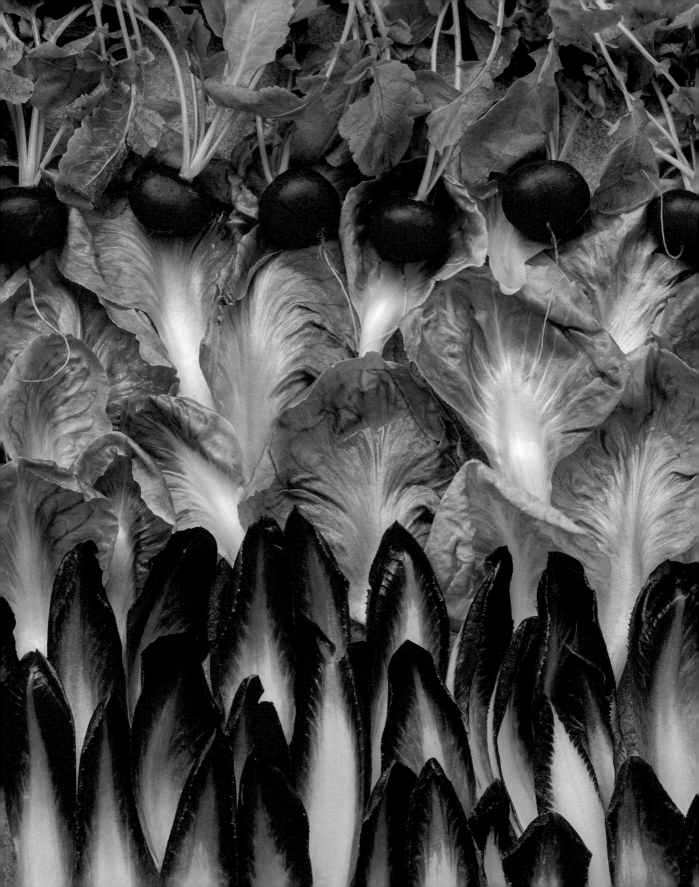

SNACKS

socca crackers

oil-free hummus

tofu pizza bites

peanut butter cacao nib muesli bars

raw cacao hemp seed bliss balls

cashew lemon dip

chocolate chickpea dip

nut-free bliss balls

socca crackers

75 g/¾ cup gram/chickpea flour
5 g/1 tablespoon nutritional yeast
½ teaspoon sea salt
¼ teaspoon garlic powder
¼ teaspoon ground cumin

baking sheet lined with parchment paper

MAKES ABOUT 25 CRACKERS

Preheat the oven to 200°C (400°F) Gas 6.

In a bowl, combine all the ingredients together with 200 ml/1 cup water using a whisk to remove any lumps.

Pour the mixture onto the baking sheet, spreading it out in an even layer, and bake in the preheated oven for 25–30 minutes. After 20 minutes of cooking, take the socca flatbread out of the oven and slice it into crackers using a sharp knife before flipping them and placing them back onto the baking sheet. Return to the oven to crisp up for 5–10 minutes. Remove from the oven and leave to cool.

Store in an airtight container.

oil-free hummus

1 x 420-g/15-oz. can chickpeas
1 lemon
2 tablespoons tahini
½ teaspoon garlic powder
½ teaspoon onion powder
½ teaspoon sea salt

SERVES 4–6

Drain and rinse the chickpeas, then add all of the ingredients to a food processor with 60 ml/¼ cup water and blend until creamy and smooth.

Store in an airtight container in the fridge for up to 1 week.

Variations: add basil, sun-dried tomatoes, cumin seeds, more garlic or cooked beetroot.

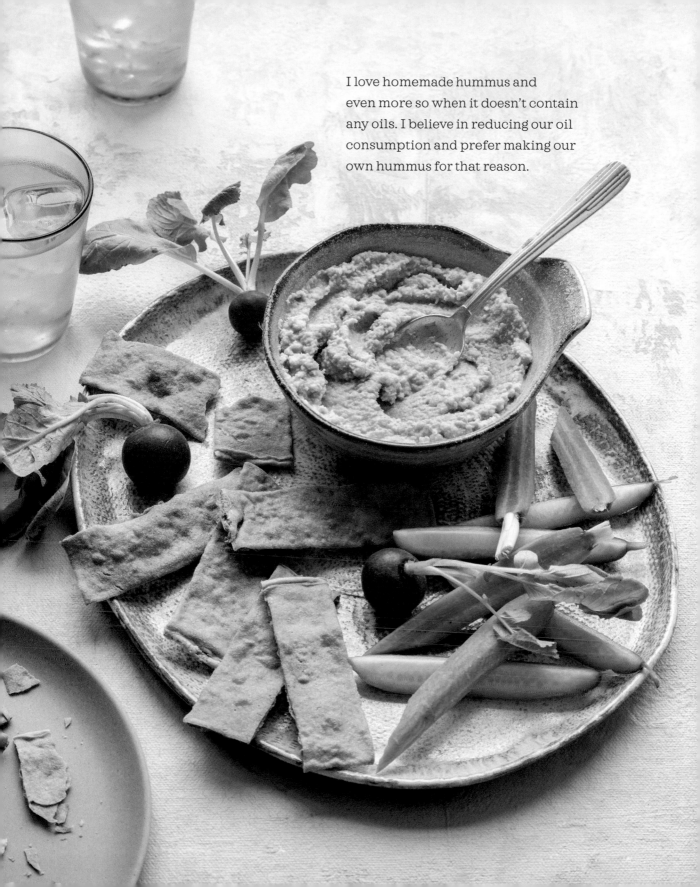

I love homemade hummus and even more so when it doesn't contain any oils. I believe in reducing our oil consumption and prefer making our own hummus for that reason.

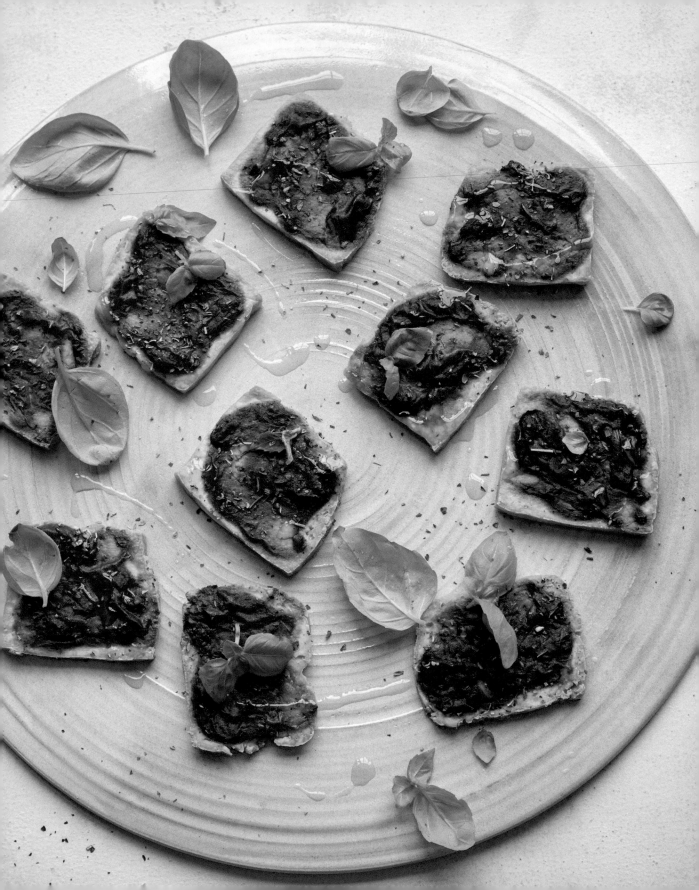

tofu pizza bites

Tofu is a great plant-based source of protein and calcium and a must in a healthy vegan diet. This recipe is a winning lunch or snack to pack for your kids' lunchboxes as it is a great way to add tofu and protein into their day. And who doesn't love pizza? These tofu pizza bites would also make a good platter for a party or when entertaining.

450 g/1 lb. extra firm tofu
60 ml/¼ cup passata/strained
   tomatoes or pizza paste
½ teaspoon onion powder
1 teaspoon dried Italian herbs
small handful of basil leaves

*baking sheet lined with parchment
   paper*

MAKES 10 PIZZA BITES

PREP TIME: 10 MINUTES
COOKING TIME: 25–30 MINUTES

Preheat the oven to 200°C (400°F) Gas 6.

Drain the tofu and press down on the (covered) tofu with heavy books or pans and chopping boards to remove the excess water. Pat it dry with paper towels, then slice the tofu into slices about 5-mm/¼-inch thick.

Lay the tofu slices on the lined baking sheet, top with a small spoonful of passata/strained tomatoes or pizza paste and spread with the spoon.

Sprinkle the onion powder and dried Italian herbs over the top and bake in the preheated oven for 25–30 minutes. Top with basil leaves and serve warm.

peanut butter cacao nib muesli bars

200 g/2 cups quick oats
140 g/½ cup plus 2 tablespoons
  smooth peanut butter
80 ml/⅓ cup maple syrup
60 g/½ cup cacao nibs

*brownie pan lined with parchment
  paper*

MAKES 12 BARS

**PREP TIME: 10 MINUTES
PLUS 1 HOUR CHILLING TIME**

Combine all the ingredients together in a mixing bowl, making sure to coat the oats with peanut butter.

Spoon the mixture into the prepared brownie pan and press down the muesli mixture firmly and evenly with your fingers or a spatula.

Leave to set in the fridge for 1 hour.

Remove from the fridge and into cut bars before serving. Store in an airtight container in the fridge.

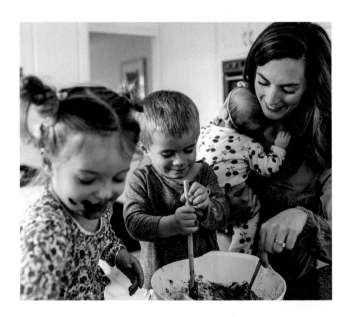

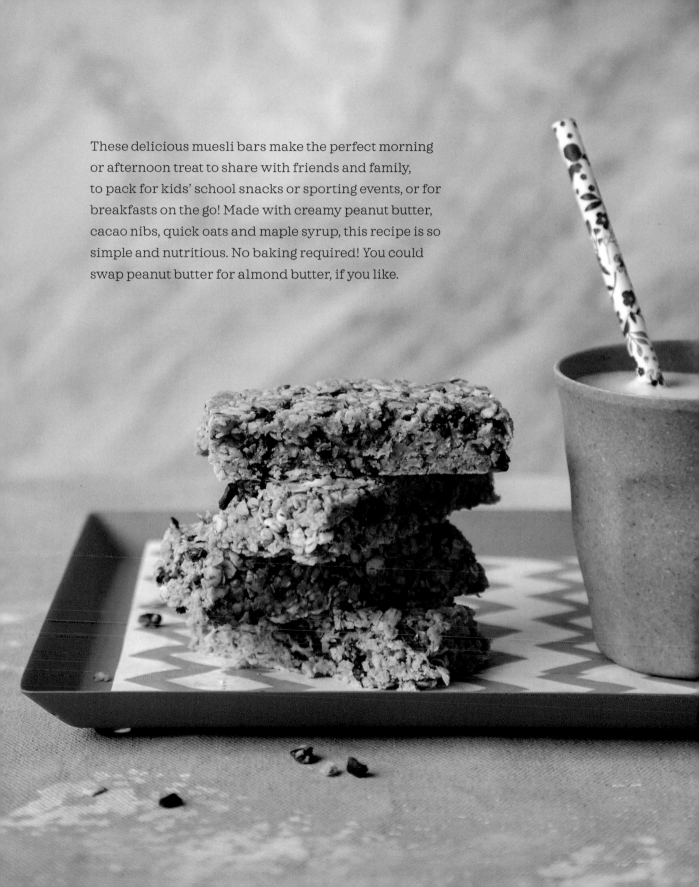

These delicious muesli bars make the perfect morning or afternoon treat to share with friends and family, to pack for kids' school snacks or sporting events, or for breakfasts on the go! Made with creamy peanut butter, cacao nibs, quick oats and maple syrup, this recipe is so simple and nutritious. No baking required! You could swap peanut butter for almond butter, if you like.

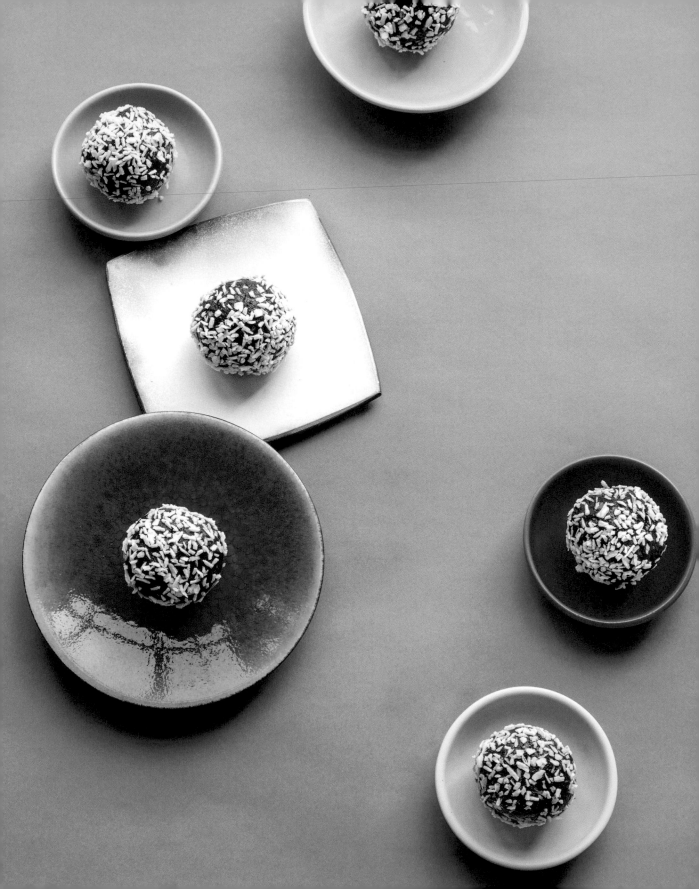

raw cacao hemp seed bliss balls

I love making bliss balls and adding extra nutrition with hemp seeds. These make the best snacks when I need a pick-me-up or crave some chocolate. If you don't have hemp seeds, you can sub with sunflower seeds, coconut flour or extra nuts. These bliss balls can be frozen or stored in the fridge. They make the perfect healthy treat to share with friends or as part of your healthy weekly meal planning.

140 g/1 cup pitted dates
150 g/1 cup raw cashews
   or almonds
20 g/3 tablespoons raw cacao
   powder
40 g/⅓ cup hemp seeds, plus
   extra to coat
desiccated/dried shredded
   coconut, to coat

MAKES 12–16 BLISS BALLS

PREP TIME: 10 MINUTES

In a food processor or high-speed blender, blitz the dates and nuts together until finely chopped.

Add in the cacao powder, hemp seeds and blend further.

Add in 1½ tablespoons water, a little at a time, to make the dough sticky.

Divide and roll the dough into 12–16 balls with your hands, then roll them in desiccated coconut, extra seeds or leave uncoated as they are.

Store them in an airtight container in the fridge for up to 1 week.

cashew lemon dip

150 g/1 cup raw cashews, soaked in cold water
   for 3–6 hours
2–3 tablespoons maple syrup
2–3 tablespoons almond milk
½ teaspoon vanilla essence
juice 1 lemon

SERVES 4

**PREP TIME: 5 MINUTES, PLUS SOAKING TIME,
& CHILLING 1 HOUR**

Rinse and drain the soaked cashews.

Blend the cashews and all the remaining
ingredients together in a high-speed blender
until creamy. Then pour the mixture into a
bowl and leave to chill in the fridge for 1 hour.

Serve and use as a dip for fruit.

Store in an airtight container in the fridge for
up to 3 days.

chocolate chickpea dip

1 x 400-g/14-oz. can salt-free chickpeas
   (or rinse them very well)
25 g/¼ cup raw cacao powder
60 ml/¼ cup maple syrup
60 ml/¼ cup coconut cream or coconut milk
1 teaspoon vanilla essence

SERVES 4

PREP TIME: 5 MINUTES

Drain and thoroughly rinse the canned
chickpeas.

Add the chickpeas to a blender or food
processor.

Add in all the remaining ingredients and blend
until creamy, scraping the side of the blender
or food processor if needed.

Serve in a bowl with fruit, bananas, crackers,
pancakes or biscuits to dip.

I often use blended cashews to make vegan cheese or raw vegan cheesecakes, but I also like this simple sweet cashew lemon dip to serve with fruits, granola, with a slice of cake or as it is!

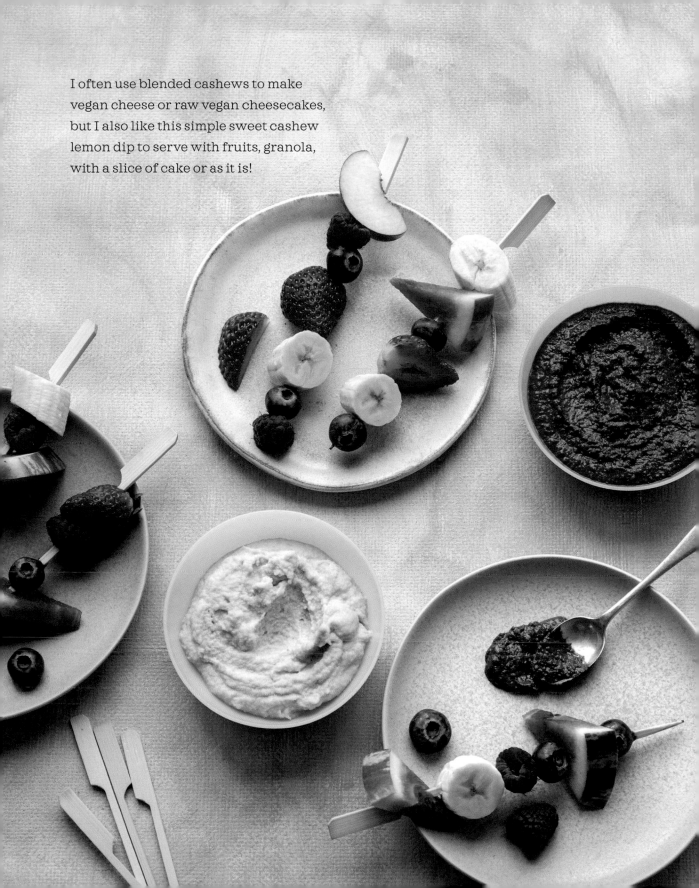

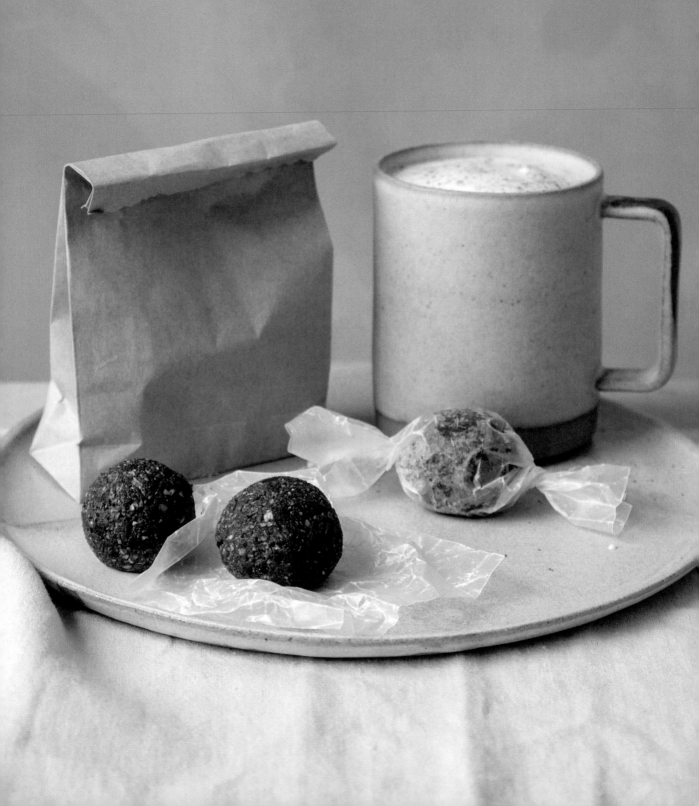

nut-free bliss balls

I know how hard it is to find easy healthy snacks to pack for school
lunchboxes, and snacks that are nut-free now that the nut-free policy
is in place in most schools and day care centres. That's why I created
these super-easy nut-free bliss balls. They only require two ingredients
and can be made with lots of different flavours to customize them.

10 Medjool dates, pitted (about
    140 g/5 oz. pitted weight)
100 g/1 cup rolled/old-fashioned
    oats

OPTIONAL INGREDIENTS
2 tablespoons raw cacao powder
1 teaspoon vanilla extract
grated orange zest, to taste
peppermint oil, to taste
1 teaspoon ground cinnamon
½ teaspoon sea salt

MAKES 12 BLISS BALLS

PREP TIME: 10 MINUTES

In a high-speed blender or food processor, combine
the dates and the oats and blend together until finely
chopped.

Add in 2 tablespoons water and pulse until sticky.

Add in your choice of optional ingredients to change
up the flavour and blend to combine.

Divide and roll the mixture into 12 bliss balls with your
hands and then store in an airtight container the fridge
for a few days.

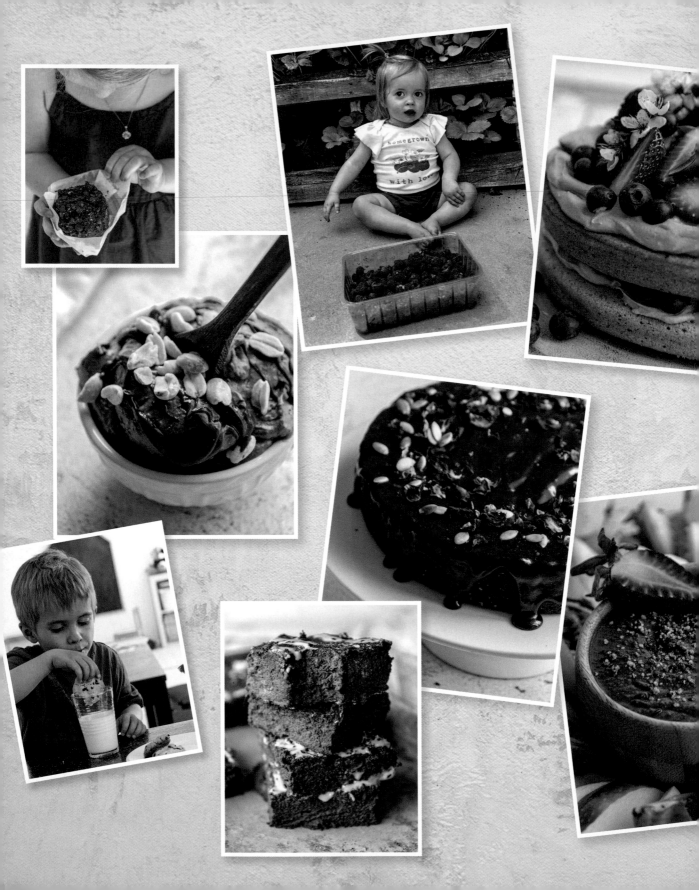

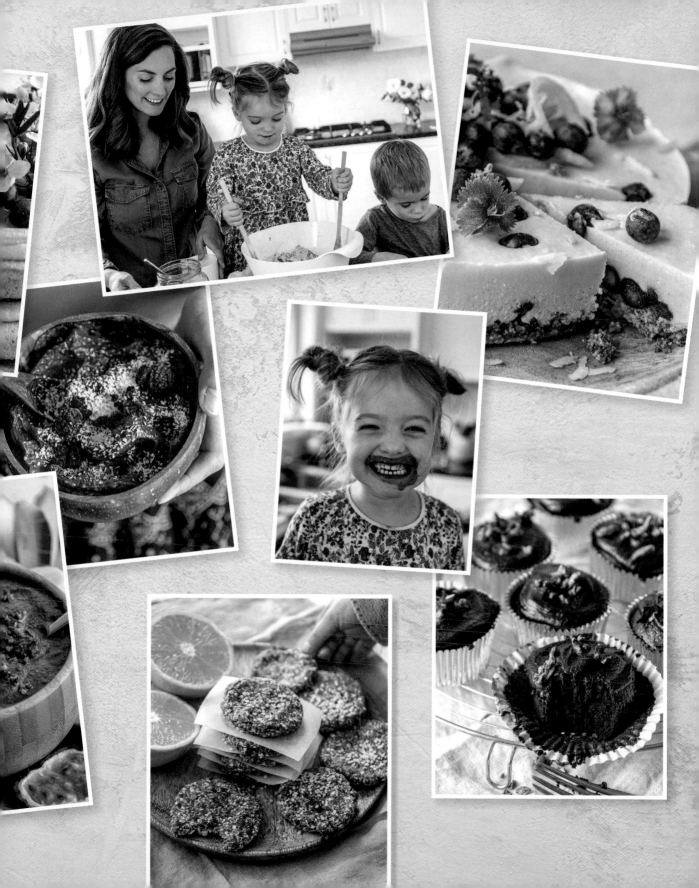

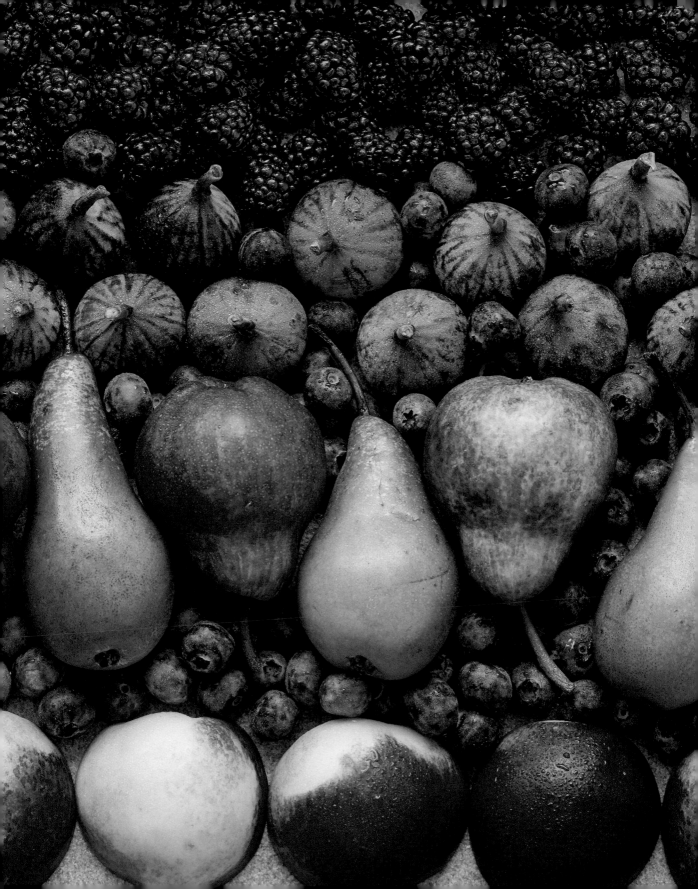

DESSERT

'nana nice cream 3 ways

mango coconut popsicles

oat banana bread

fudgy sweet potato tahini brownies

chocolate mud cupcakes

beetroot chocolate cake

raw blueberry & lemon cashew cheesecake

peanut butter cacao nib cookies

raw orange & hemp seed cookies

sweet potato, apple & cinnamon muffins

chocolate chip courgette muffins

almond tahini coconut cups

superfood coconut sprinkles

avocado banana chocolate mousse

fruit-sweetened birthday cake with berry coconut icing

'nana nice cream 3 ways

Making 'ice cream'-like desserts using frozen bananas is probably one of the best healthy recipes out there! Vegan ice cream with no added funny ingredients and made from wholesome natural bananas – if you haven't tried it, I highly recommend you freeze your next lot of ripe bananas and use them to make one of my 'nana nice cream recipes. A big hit with little kids and big kids at heart!

neopolitan

5 medium-sized frozen (peeled)
  bananas
60 ml/¼ cup coconut milk
1 teaspoon vanilla extract
30 g/¼ cup raw cacao powder
150 g/1 cup frozen strawberries

PREP TIME: 5 MINUTES

SERVES 2–3

In a food processor or high-speed blender, combine the bananas and coconut milk together for a few minutes until the bananas turn into a creamy frozen ice cream.

Spoon two-thirds of the ice cream into two separate bowls. Keep one third in the blender.

In one bowl, combine the banana ice cream with the vanilla extract. In the other bowl, stir the cacao powder into the banana ice cream.

Blend the frozen strawberries with the remaining third of the banana ice cream until creamy.

Spoon the chocolate ice cream into a large glass bowl, then add the vanilla ice cream followed by the strawberry ice cream. Return the bowl to the freezer for 30 minutes if the ice cream has melted a little too much before serving.

chocolate peanut butter

3 medium-sized frozen (peeled)
   bananas
60 ml/¼ cup coconut milk
60 ml/¼ cup smooth peanut
   butter
30 g/¼ cup raw cacao powder
peanut butter, peanuts and
   chocolate sauce, to top
   (optional)

PREP TIME: 5 MINUTES

SERVES 2–3

DF EF GF WF
OF SYF

In a food processor or high-speed blender, combine all the ingredients together for a few minutes until the bananas turn into a creamy frozen ice cream.

Spoon the ice cream into bowls and top with extra peanut butter, peanuts and/or chocolate sauce.

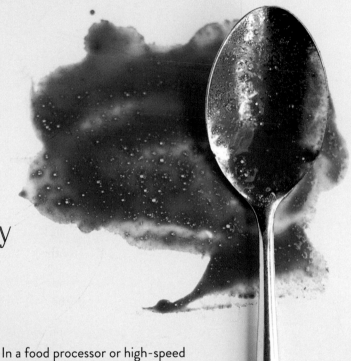

coconut & raspberry

3 medium-sized frozen (peeled)
   bananas
60 ml/¼ cup coconut milk
150 g/1 cup frozen raspberries
20 g/¼ cup desiccated/dried
   shredded coconut
extra desiccated coconut and
   raspberries, to top (optional)

PREP TIME: 5 MINUTES

SERVES 2–3

DF EF GF WF
NF OF SF SYF

In a food processor or high-speed blender, combine all the ingredients together for a few minutes until the bananas turn into a creamy frozen ice cream.

Spoon into bowls and enjoy with toppings, if desired.

mango coconut popsicles

Summertime in Australia really is the best. We are so lucky to have delicious sweet mangoes all summer long. My family and I make the most of the mango season and when we have a few too many ripe mangoes I make these delicious, easy and refreshing mango coconut popsicles to enjoy on hot summer afternoons. I love knowing exactly what is in my kids' ice-creams. No fillers and only three ingredients! You could even leave out the maple syrup if you are using very sweet ripe mangoes. I sometimes add a passion fruit or two after blending the mango to change the flavour.

2 ripe mangoes, peeled, pitted and diced
1 x 400-ml/14-fl. oz. can coconut cream
1 tablespoon maple syrup

6 popsicle moulds

MAKES 6

PREP TIME: 5 MINUTES
FREEZING TIME: 6 HOURS OR OVERNIGHT

Blend the mango, coconut cream and maple syrup together in a blender or food processor until smooth and creamy.

Pour into each popsicle mould. Put the moulds (upright) in the freezer for a minimum of 4–6 hours or overnight before serving.

Remove the moulds by running them under warm water briefly. You can store the popsicles in an airtight container in the freezer after removing the moulds to enjoy them later on.

Optional: Add vanilla extract and passion fruit.

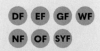

fudgy sweet potato tahini brownies

I have been making these super-healthy, fudgy sweet potato brownies for the past 5 years. I make them every time I have new friends or guests coming over. They are really easy to make and taste delicious warm or eaten cold straight from the fridge the next day. I find it hard to stop at just one piece! I tend to use leftover roasted sweet potatoes for this recipe or I cook the sweet potatoes the night before I want to make the brownies.

450 g/16 oz. sweet potatoes, peeled
125 ml/½ cup almond milk
75 g/½ cup buckwheat flour or plain/all-purpose gluten-free flour
65 g/⅔ cup almond meal
70 g/½ cup coconut sugar
6 tablespoons raw cacao powder or cocoa powder
40 ml/⅓ cup tahini
½ teaspoon vanilla extract
pinch of salt

TAHINI SAUCE
40 ml/⅓ cup tahini
2 tablespoons raw cacao powder
1 tablespoon melted coconut oil
1 tablespoon maple syrup

brownie pan, lined with parchment paper

SERVES 9–12

PREP TIME: 15 MINUTES
COOKING TIME: 30–40 MINUTES

Steam, roast or boil the sweet potatoes, drain and leave to cool.

Preheat the oven to 180°C (350°F) Gas 4.

In a food processor combine the cooked sweet potatoes with all the remaining ingredients. Mix until well combined and all the lumps are gone.

Spoon the mixture into the prepared brownie pan and smooth over with a spoon.

Bake in the preheated oven for 30–40 minutes or until a knife inserted comes out clean. Allow to cool slightly.

Meanwhile, to make the tahini sauce, combine all the ingredients together in a bowl and mix until smooth.

When the brownies have cooled slightly, drizzle over the tahini sauce and slice the brownies into squares.

The brownies can be stored in the fridge in an airtight container for up to 1 week.

oat banana bread

This moist and super-healthy banana bread is a real favourite
in our home. Made with ripe mashed bananas and oat flour it is a
winning healthy vegan treat. It is also nut-free and suitable for school
lunchboxes. We love it warm from the oven as an afternoon treat or
cold the next day. If you do not have oat flour, you can make your own
by blending oats in a high-speed blender, or alternatively you could
use buckwheat flour.

3 large ripe bananas
240 g/2 cups oat flour
1 teaspoon vanilla extract
1 teaspoon baking powder
35 g/¼ cup coconut sugar
250 ml/1 cup coconut or oat milk

*loaf pan, lined with parchment
   paper*

MAKES 1 LOAF

PREP TIME: 10 MINUTES
COOKING TIME: 50 MINUTES

Preheat the oven to 180°C (350°F) Gas 4.

Peel and mash the bananas in a large mixing bowl.
Add the oat flour, vanilla extract, baking powder and
sugar and combine together.

Stir in the coconut or oat milk until combined, then
pour the mixture into the prepared loaf pan.

Bake in the preheated oven for 50 minutes until
a skewer inserted into the middle comes out clean.
Leave to cool on a wire rack before slicing to serve.

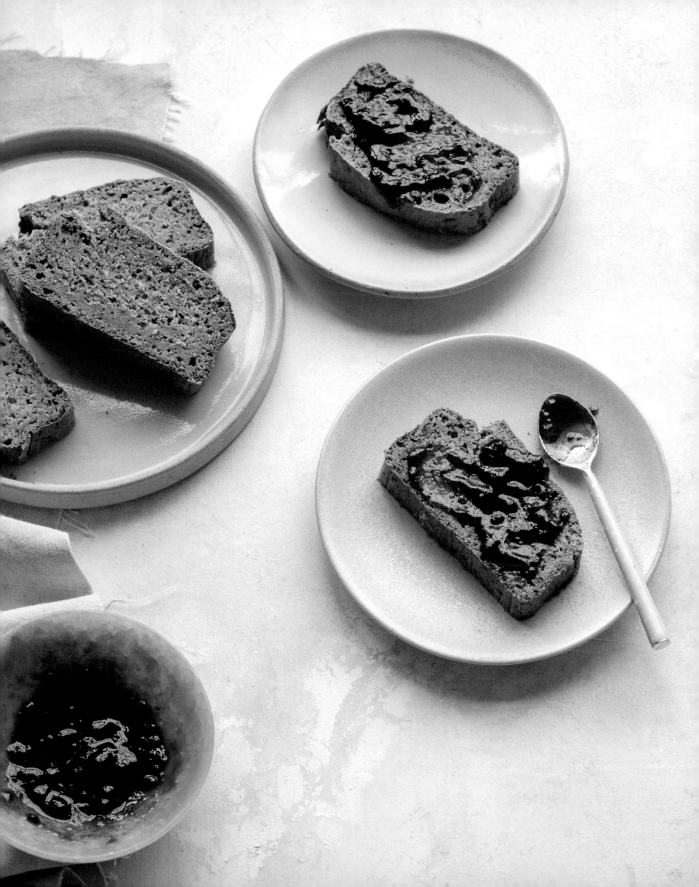

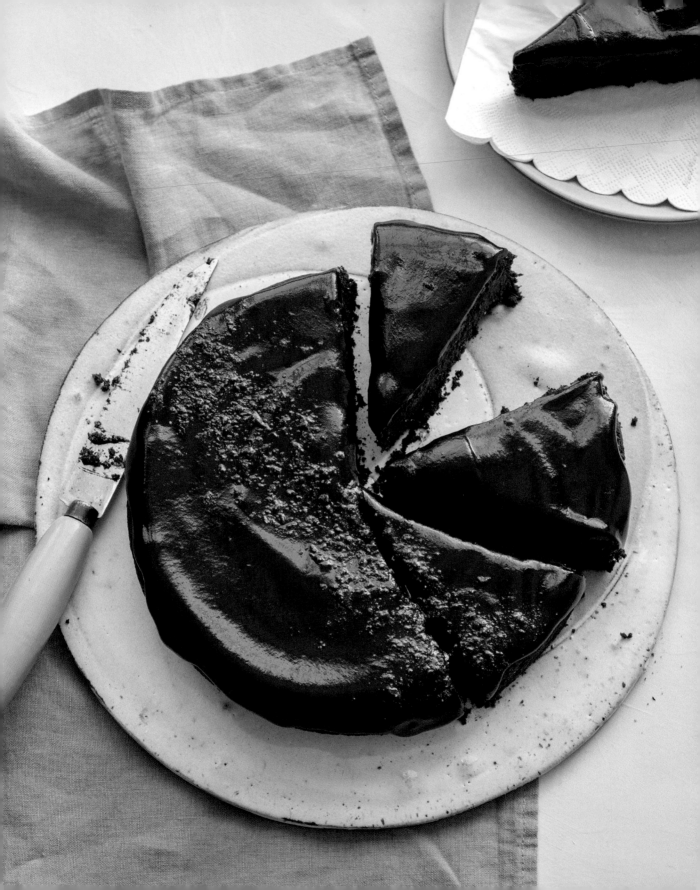

beetroot chocolate cake

This is a bit of a twist on the traditional chocolate cake with the addition of cooked beetroot, which makes this chocolate cake extra moist and delicious. This cake is also very easy to make and could be made with children. I like topping the cake with a coconut cream chocolate ganache, but you could also eat it as it is.

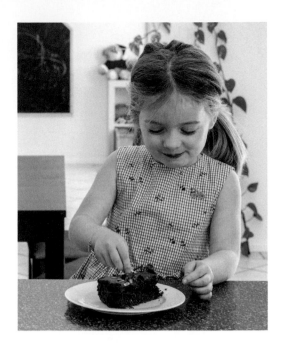

250 g/9 oz. vacuum-sealed
  cooked beetroot/beets
  (no vinegar)
2 flax eggs (2 tablespoons flaxseed
  meal and 6 tablespoons water)
225 g/1½ cups self-raising/rising
  wholemeal/whole-wheat flour
65 g/½ cup raw cacao powder
1 teaspoon vanilla extract
125 ml/½ cup maple syrup
125 ml/½ cup plant milk of choice
80 ml/⅓ cup coconut oil, melted
beetroot/beet powder, to decorate
  (optional)

CHOCOLATE GANACHE
100 g/3½ oz. dark/bittersweet
  chocolate, chopped
2 tablespoons coconut cream

*round cake pan, lined with
  parchment paper*

SERVES 9–12

PREP TIME: 10 MINUTES
COOKING TIME: 40 MINUTES

Preheat the oven to 190°C (375°F) Gas 5.

Blend or finely grate the beetroots/beets.

In a small bowl, combine the flaxseed meal with the water to create the flax eggs and leave to set on the side for 5 minutes.

In a large mixing bowl, combine the flour, cacao powder and vanilla extract. Add in the flax eggs, beetroot/beets and maple syrup and stir to combine. Add the plant milk and combine. Add the coconut oil and stir well.

Pour the cake batter into the lined cake pan and bake in the preheated oven for 40 minutes or until a skewer or a knife inserted comes out clean. Leave to cool slightly in the pan then transfer to a wire rack.

For the ganache, melt the dark/bittersweet chocolate and coconut cream in a heatproof bowl over a saucepan of simmering water. Stir until the chocolate melts and the mixture is smooth. Remove from the heat. Spread over the top of the cake and sprinkle over a little beetroot/beet powder, if desired. Serve in slices.

chocolate mud cupcakes

These cupcakes are my ultimate birthday party treat to suit anyone as they are vegan, gluten-free, nut-free and can be made with low sugar yet they still taste amazing and both children and adults alike love them! Swap the coffee for extra hot water when making them for children. And you can use wheat flour if you prefer.

1 flax egg (1 tablespoon flaxseed meal combined with 3 tablespoons water)
100 g/½ cup vegan butter
100 g/3½ oz. dark/bittersweet chocolate, chopped
125 ml/½ cup hot water
60 ml/¼ cup coffee/hot water
100–140 g/¾ cup–1 cup coconut sugar or sweetener of choice
100 g/⅔ cup plain/all-purpose gluten-free flour
40 g/¼ cup self-raising/rising gluten-free flour
2 tablespoons raw cacao powder
cacao nibs, edible flowers or sprinkles, to decorate (optional)

CHOCOLATE GANACHE
100 g/3½ oz. dark/bittersweet chocolate, chopped
2 tablespoons coconut cream

12-hole cupcake pan, lined with cupcake cases

MAKES 12

PREP TIME: 15 MINUTES
COOKING TIME: 20–25 MINUTES

Preheat the oven to 170°C (325°F) Gas 3.

In a small bowl, make the flax egg by combining the flaxseed meal and water. Leave to set for 5 minutes.

In a saucepan set over a medium heat, combine the vegan butter, chopped dark/bittersweet chocolate, hot water and coffee (or additional hot water). Stir for a few minutes until the chocolate and butter melt completely. Turn off the heat, add the sugar and stir to combine. Set aside and leave to cool slightly.

In a mixing bowl, pour in the chocolate mixture, then add the flours and cacao powder, a little at a time, stirring with a whisk. Add the flax egg and whisk until smooth.

Pour the cupcake batter into the cupcake cases almost to the top of each and bake in the preheated oven for 20–25 minutes or until cooked through. Leave to cool completely on a wire rack.

For the ganache, melt the dark/bittersweet chocolate and coconut cream in a heatproof bowl over a saucepan of simmering water. Stir until the chocolate melts and the mixture is smooth. Remove from the heat. Spread the ganache with a spoon over the top of the cupcakes and decorate with cacao nibs, flowers or sprinkles.

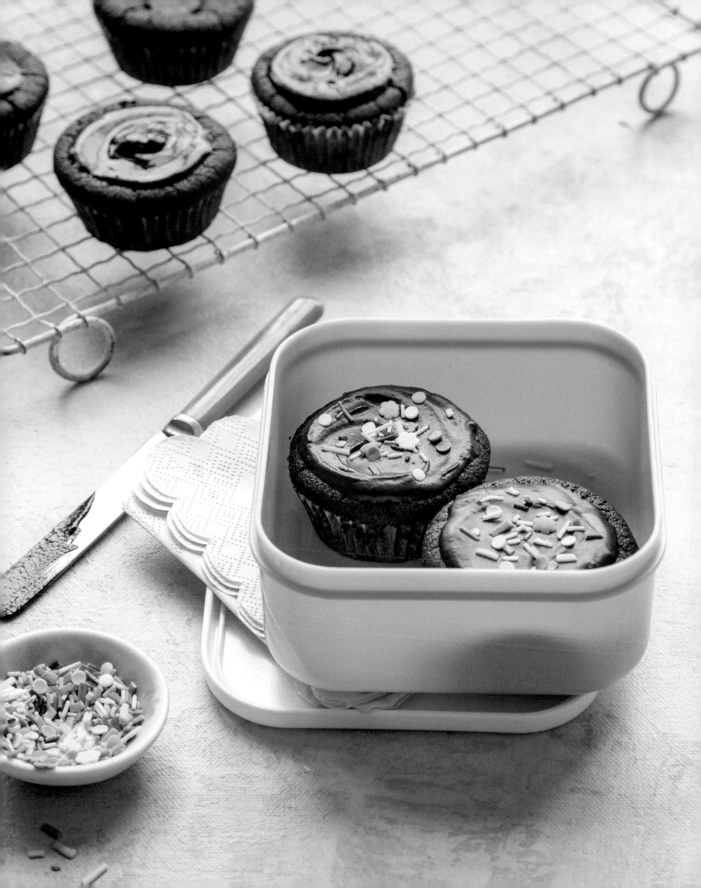

raw blueberry & lemon cashew cheesecake

I am a huge fan of raw vegan cheesecakes with a creamy cashew filling and a nutty base. I also like how easy they are to make using a food processor or high-speed blender and the fact that you can store them in the freezer. I have made so many in the past, raspberry and coconut, strawberries and cream, chocolate and hazelnuts, snickers ... but my favourite of them all is this raw blueberry and lemon cashew cheesecake. I like adding a tablespoon of nutritional yeast to add a 'cheese' taste to the cheesecake, but feel free to leave it out.

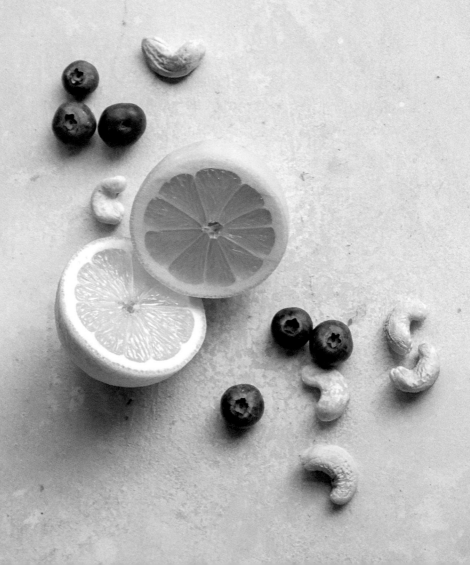

BASE
150 g/1 cup raw almonds
150 g/1 cup pitted dates
45 g/½ cup desiccated/dried
   shredded coconut

BLUEBERRY & LEMON CASHEW FILLING
125 g/1 cup frozen or fresh
   blueberries, plus extra to top
   and decorate
300 g/2 cups raw cashews (soaked
   in cold water for 2–3 hours, or
   for 10 minutes in boiling water)
125 ml/½ cup coconut cream
2 tablespoons melted coconut oil
85 ml/⅓ cup maple syrup
1 teaspoon vanilla extract
zest and juice of 1 lemon or
   10 drops of food-grade lemon
   essential oil
1 tablespoon nutritional yeast

*cake pan, lined with long strips
   of parchment paper*

SERVES 9–12

PREP TIME: 15 MINUTES
SOAKING TIME: 2–3 HOURS
OR OVERNIGHT
FREEZING TIME: 2–3 HOURS

DF EF GF WF
SYF

Line the cake pan with strips of parchment paper (this will be used to help remove the cheesecake from the pan later).

To make the base, blend the almonds in a high-speed blender or food processor until finely chopped. Add the dates and desiccated/dried shredded coconut and blend until it becomes a sticky, chunky mixture. Add 1 tablespoon water, a little at a time, to help make it stick.

Transfer the base to the prepared cake pan. Press down firmly and evenly with a glass or your hands.

Spread the frozen or fresh blueberries on top of the base and place it in the freezer until set.

For the remaining filling, drain and rinse the soaked cashews, then add to a clean blender or food processor along with the coconut cream, coconut oil, maple syrup, vanilla extract, lemon and nutritional yeast and blend until smooth and creamy.

Remove the base from the freezer and pour the lemon cashew filling on top of the blueberries, spreading it evenly and carefully. Top with a few more blueberries and return it to the freezer to set for 2–3 hours.

Remove from the freezer 20–30 minutes before serving. Top with extra blueberries. Remove from the pan and serve in slices.

Store leftovers in an airtight container in the fridge for up to 2–3 days or in the freezer for 2–3 weeks.

peanut butter cacao nib cookies

I have made these cookies so many times! They are loved by both little and big kids. Chewy and crunchy, so quick to make and very low in sugar. These cookies are also gluten-free and don't require much cooking time so they are the perfect treat! Feel free to swap the cacao nibs for vegan chocolate chips, or swap the peanut butter for tahini to make them nut-free. Also delicious with a cold glass of plant milk.

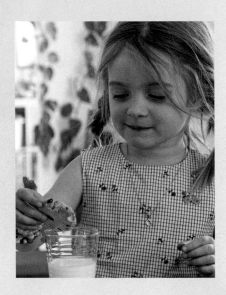

100 g/1 cup almond meal
40 g/¼ cup buckwheat flour or plain/all-purpose gluten-free flour
½ teaspoon vanilla extract
½ teaspoon baking powder
2 tablespoons melted coconut oil
65 g/¼ cup peanut butter
2 tablespoons maple syrup

2 tablespoons cacao nibs or vegan chocolate chips

baking sheet, lined with parchment paper

MAKES 10

PREP TIME: 5 MINUTES
COOKING TIME: 10 MINUTES

Preheat the oven to 180°C (350°F) Gas 4.

In a mixing bowl, combine the almond meal, buckwheat or gluten-free flour, vanilla extract and baking powder. Add the melted coconut oil, peanut butter and maple syrup and mix together well. Add in the cacao nibs or chocolate chips and stir them through the cookie dough.

Shape into 10 golf ball-sized balls of cookie dough, place them on the lined baking sheet, spaced apart and flatten them with your fingers or a fork to shape them into cookies.

Bake in the preheated oven for 10 minutes until cooked. Remove from the oven and allow to cool on a wire rack.

raw orange & hemp seed cookies

My go-to nut-free cookie recipe to serve at playdates and pack for school lunchboxes. They are super-nutritious with added vitamin C from the orange juice and zest, and iron, zinc and omega-3s from the hemp seeds. You can swap the oats for quinoa flakes and the hemp seeds for sunflower seeds, if required.

280 g/2 cups pitted dates
150 g/1½ cups rolled/old-
    fashioned oats
65 g/½ cup hemp seeds
zest and juice from 1 orange
1 teaspoon vanilla extract

MAKES 14

PREP TIME: 10 MINUTES

In a food processor, combine the dates and oats and blend together until finely chopped. Add the hemp seeds, orange zest and juice and vanilla extract and pulse until well combined and sticky.

Divide and roll the mixture into 14 balls with your hands and lay them on a tray or plate before flattening them with your fingers to form cookie shapes.

Leave to set in the fridge.

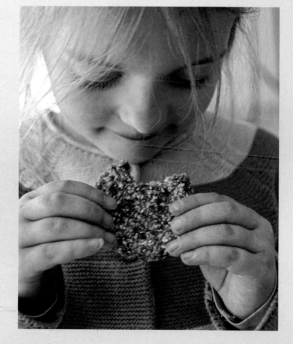

sweet potato, apple & cinnamon muffins

These muffins taste like autumn in a bite. Packed with grated sweet potato and apple for sweetness, these are a perfect treat to share on a cosy afternoon with friends and a cup of tea or chai. As well as tasting delicious, these muffins are also very nutritious as sweet potatoes are high in vitamin A, fibre, minerals and other vitamins. Also buckwheat flour is a great wholegrain flour and is gluten-free as well as being high in fibre, protein, zinc and other minerals.

300 g/2 cups buckwheat flour
1 teaspoon baking powder
70 g/½ cup coconut sugar
1 teaspoon ground cinnamon
pinch of ground nutmeg (optional)
pinch of ground all spices
    (optional)
pinch of ground ginger (optional)
2 tablespoons flaxseed meal
250 ml/1 cup oat milk
60 ml/¼ cup melted coconut oil
200 g/1 cup grated sweet potatoes
250 g/1 cup grated apples

12-hole muffin pan, lined with
    muffin cases

MAKES 12 MUFFINS

PREP TIME: 10–15 MINUTES
COOKING TIME: 40–45 MINUTES

Preheat the oven to 185°C (365°F) Gas 4½

In a bowl, combine the flour, baking powder, coconut sugar and spices and stir. Add in the flaxseed meal and oat milk and stir. Pour in the melted coconut oil and stir to combine. Add the grated sweet potatoes and apples and fold to combine with a spatula. It might take a few minutes to combine fully, but keep stirring.

Spoon the muffin batter into the paper cases in the pan until each one is half-full, then bake in the preheated oven for 40–45 minutes or until a skewer inserted in the centre comes out clean. Remove from the oven and transfer to a wire rack. Enjoy warm or cold.

Store in an airtight container for up to 3 days.

Variations: Swap the sweet potato for pumpkin or carrots. You can also add sultanas or crushed nuts and remove or add extra spices, depending on preference.

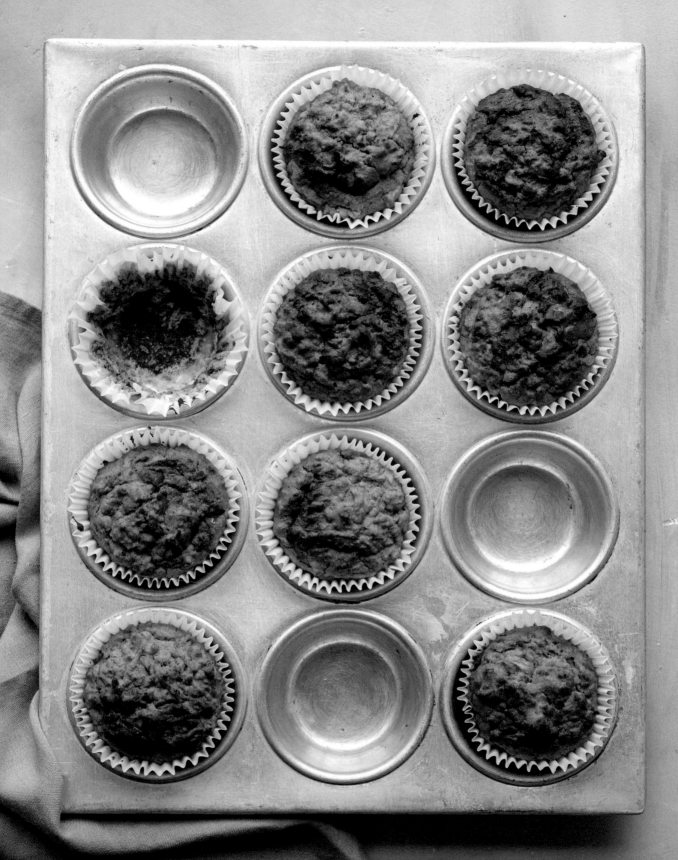

My twins absolutely love these muffins and I am more than happy to treat them to one of my healthy homemade chocolate courgette muffins. They are rich, super chocolatey and refined sugar-free. Courgettes are great for adding to baked goods due to their subtle flavour and they blend in perfectly in sweet treats. They make these muffins nice and moist and help keep added fats and oil to a minimum.

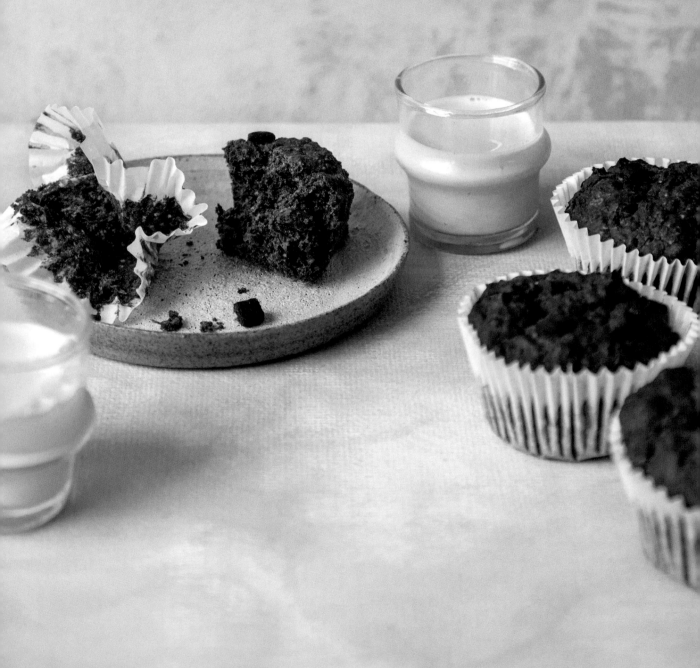

chocolate chip courgette muffins

150 g/1 cup self-raising/rising wholemeal/whole-wheat flour

150 g/1 cup wholemeal/whole-wheat plain/all-purpose flour

65 g/½ cup raw cacao powder

70 g/½ cup coconut sugar

2 tablespoons flaxseed meal

250 ml/1 cup oat milk

1 medium-sized courgette/zucchini, grated

125 ml/½ cup melted coconut oil

75 g/½ cup dairy-free chocolate chips, plus extra to decorate

12-hole muffin pan, lined with muffin cases

MAKES 12

PREP TIME: 10 MINUTES
COOKING TIME: 25–30 MINUTES

Preheat the oven to 180°C (350°F) Gas 4.

In a mixing bowl, combine the flours together, then add the cacao powder, coconut sugar and flaxseed meal and combine well. Add the oat milk and stir to combine.

Add the grated courgette/zucchini to the muffin batter. Fold and combine well. Add in the melted coconut oil and stir to combine, then fold in the chocolate chips.

Spoon the muffin batter into the paper muffin cases about halfway to the top. If desired, sprinkle a few extra chocolate chips on the top. Bake in the preheated oven for 25–30 minutes or until a skewer inserted in the centre comes out clean. Remove from the oven and allow to cool on a wire rack.

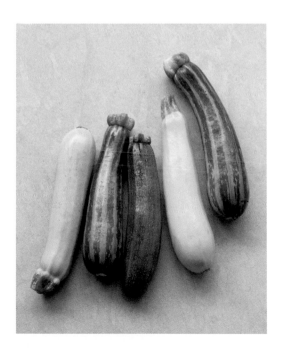

DF EF

NF

almond tahini coconut cups

Raw energy desserts like these almond tahini coconut cups are great nutritious treats for vegan kids. My family and I go crazy for them! High in calcium from the tahini, almonds and hemp seeds, they are also gluten-free and refined sugar-free. You can store them in the freezer. My freezer always contains half a batch to share with unexpected visitors.

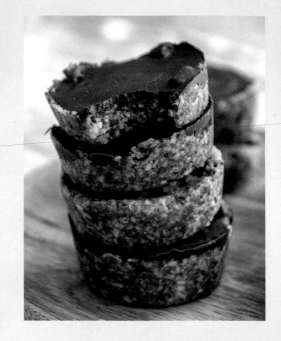

240 g/1½ cups raw almonds
65 g/½ cup hemp seeds
135 g/1½ cups desiccated/dried
   shredded coconut
35 g/¼ cup pitted dates
60 ml/¼ cup maple syrup
40 ml/⅓ cup tahini
1 teaspoon flaxseed meal
50 g/2 oz. dark/bittersweet
   chocolate, chopped

12–15 silicone muffin moulds

MAKES 12–15

PREP TIME: 15 MINUTES
CHILLING TIME: 1–2 HOURS

In a food processor, combine the almonds, hemp seeds and coconut and process until fine. Add in the dates, maple syrup, tahini and flaxseed meal and process until it forms a sticky dough. Add 1 tablespoon water and blend further if not sticky enough.

Divide and press the sticky dough into the silicone muffin moulds.

Melt the dark/bittersweet chocolate in a heatproof bowl set over a pan of simmering water. Pour the melted chocolate on top of each of the almond tahini cups. Put the moulds in the fridge and leave to set for a few hours. Press out of the moulds and serve.

Store in an airtight container in the fridge or freezer.

superfood coconut sprinkles

I prefer making my own healthy superfood sprinkles for my children to avoid excess sugars, artificial colours, waxing and flavourings usually found in sprinkles. My superfood coconut sprinkles can be used to top cakes, yogurt, ice cream, chocolate and fruit salads. I used turmeric, beetroot/beet and matcha powder, but you could also use spirulina, dragon fruit powder, blue algae or other superfood powders.

90 g/1 cup desiccated/
dried shredded coconut
½ teaspoon ground
turmeric
½ teaspoon beetroot/beet
powder

½ teaspoon matcha
powder

MAKES 1 CUP

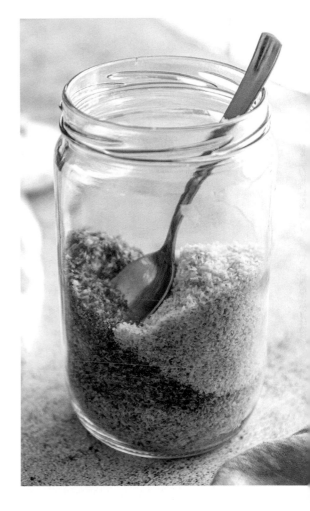

In small separate bowls, combine one third of the desiccated/dried shredded coconut with ½ teaspoon each of the superfood powders and stir to combine the powder with the coconut.

Store in an airtight jar either combining them together or keeping them separately.

Variations: You can use dragon fruit, raw cacao, blue algae and/or spirulina powders to make other colours.

avocado banana chocolate mousse

I have been making this avocado chocolate mousse for years now.
It satisfies any chocolate mousse cravings while being made from
vegan wholefoods. Packed with good fats, fibre and antioxidants and
being refined sugar-free it is really delicious and healthy. Best served
cold from the fridge or the mousse can also be made as a substitute
for chocolate icing/frosting on cakes!

3 medium-sized ripe bananas,
    peeled
flesh from 2 medium-sized ripe
    avocados
30 g/¼ cup raw cacao powder
60 ml/¼ cup maple syrup
1 teaspoon vanilla extract
berries and crushed nuts, to serve

SERVES 3–4

PREP TIME: 5 MINUTES
CHILLING TIME: 1 HOUR

In a blender, combine all the ingredients together
and blend until smooth and creamy.

Spoon into 3–4 small bowls and place in the fridge
to chill or enjoy straight away.

Add berries and crushed nuts, to serve.

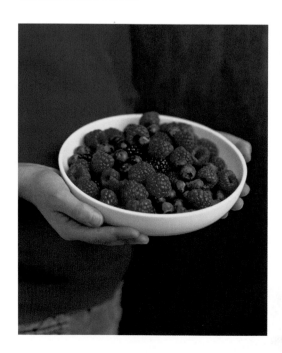

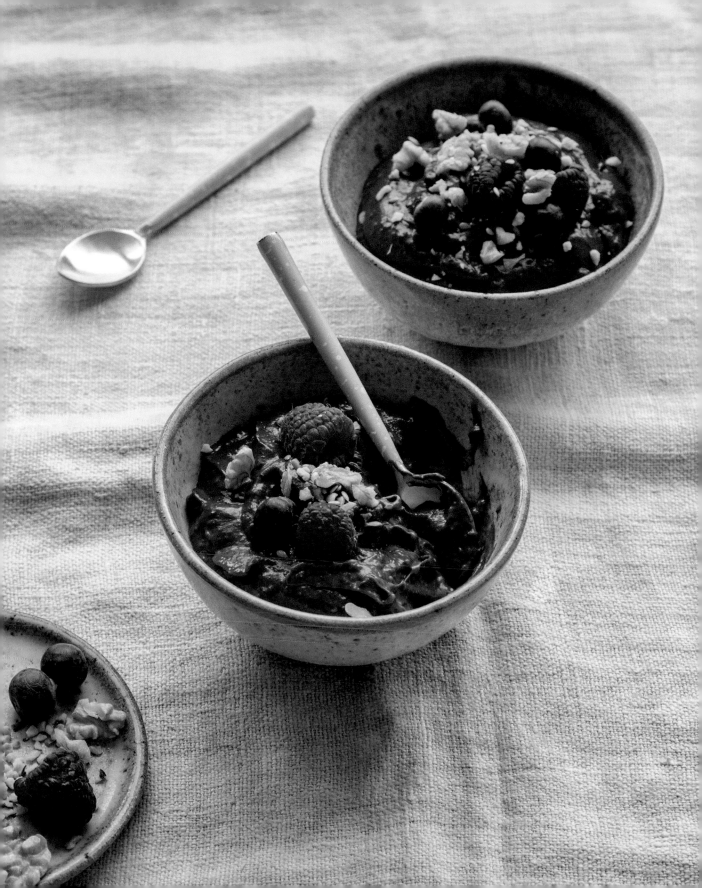

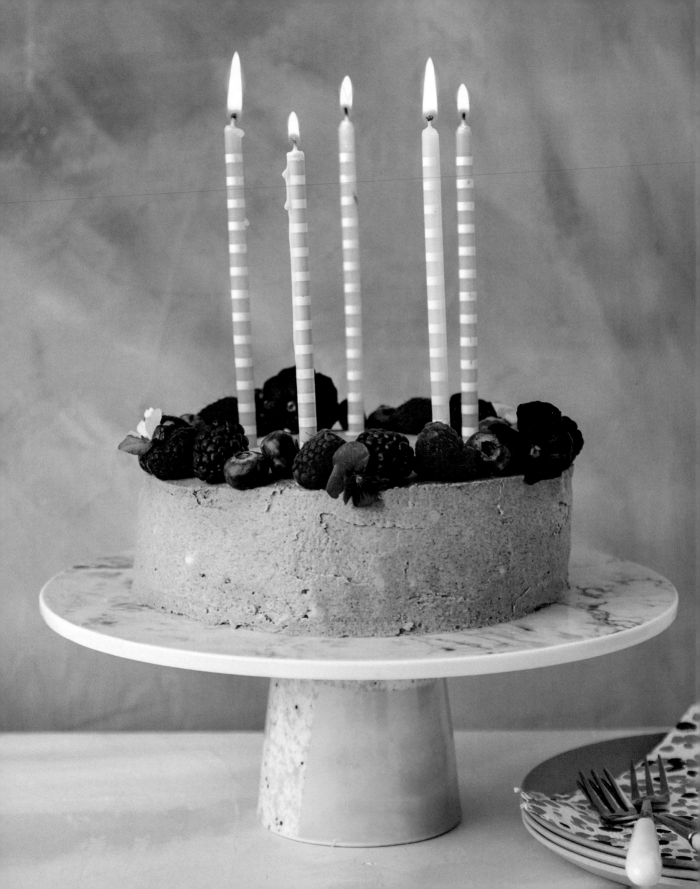

fruit-sweetened birthday cake with berry coconut icing

This is probably the healthiest birthday cake out there! I made this special cake for my daughter Annabelle's first birthday. It is really delicious as well as very easy to make and very allergy-friendly.

300 g/2 cups plain/all-purpose wholemeal/whole-wheat flour
1½ teaspoons baking powder
1 teaspoon vanilla extract
1 tablespoon flaxseed meal
240 g/1 cup apple purée
125 ml/½ cup oat milk or coconut milk
60 ml/¼ cup apple juice (or maple syrup/extra oat milk)
60 ml/¼ cup olive oil
berries and edible flowers, to decorate (optional)

BERRY COCONUT ICING/FROSTING
1 x 400-g/14-oz. can coconut cream, solidified in the fridge
120 g/½ cup berry and pear purée
½ teaspoon beetroot/beet powder

2 x 20-cm/8-inch round cake pans, greased with olive oil

SERVES 8–10

PREP TIME: 25 MINUTES
COOKING TIME: 25 MINUTES

Preheat the oven to 180°C (350°F) Gas 4.

In a mixing bowl, combine the flour, baking powder, vanilla extract and flaxseed meal. Pour in the apple purée and combine with a spoon. Add in the milk, apple juice and olive oil and combine well.

Pour half of the cake batter into one cake pan and the second half into the other pan; level the tops. Bake in the preheated oven for 25 minutes. Remove from the oven and allow to cool for 5 minutes before removing from the pans and allowing to cool completely on wire racks.

To make the berry coconut icing/frosting, combine the solidified coconut cream (the top layer only from the can) in a blender with the berry and pear purée and the beetroot/beet powder until smooth.

Spread one third of the berry coconut icing/frosting over the bottom cake layer with a spatula. Cover with the top cake layer and spread the remaining icing/frosting over the top and sides of the cake, covering as evenly as you can. To decorate (if desired), arrange berries, edible flowers and candles on top.

Alternatively, spread a thick layer of the berry coconut icing/frosting on top of the first cake, top with berries and place the second cake on top. Spread a thick layer of the remaining coconut icing/frosting on top of the second cake and add more berries, plus edible flowes. Serve straight away or store in an airtight container.

index

picture credits

Clare Winfield
Jacket front and back
Pages 1, 2, 3, 5, 7, 10, 11, 18, 21, 22, 24, 27, 28, 31, 32, 34, 37,
38, 39, 40, 41, 42, 43, 45, 46, 47, 48, 49, 50, 51, 52, 54,
55, 56, 57, 58, 60, 63, 64, 67, 68, 69, 71, 72, 74–75, 77,
78, 79, 81, 82/83, 85, 86, 89, 90, 92–93, 95, 96, 98, 100,
101, 102, 105, 106, 109, 110, 111, 114, 118–119, 121, 122, 125,
131, 132, 133, 137, 138, 140–141, 142–143.

Claire Power, Kristen Cunningham and Emily Ellis
Jacket spine
Pages 8–9, 20, 29, 33, 36, 44, 53, 58–59, 88, 112–113, 123,
128, 129, 134, 135.

Ed Anderson
Pages 12, 25.

Matt Russell
Page 15.

Kate Whitaker
Page 82.

Lisa Linder
Pages 117, 136.

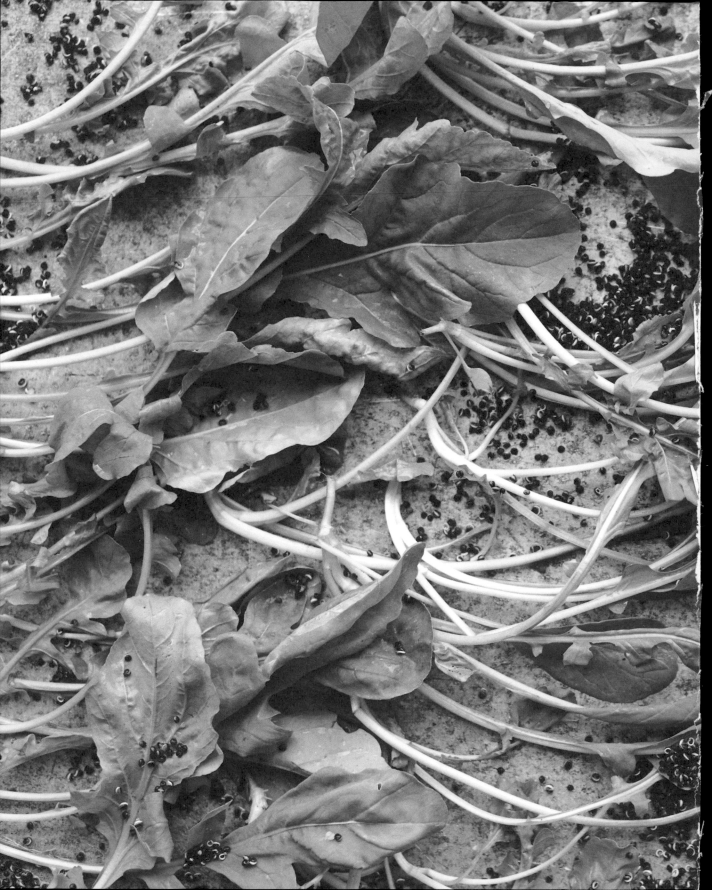